Adolescent Females' Reproductive Health in Nigeria

T0175217

European University Studies

Europäische Hochschulschriften
Publications Universitaires Européennes

Series XXII
Sociology

Reihe XXII Série XXII
Soziologie
Sociologie

Vol./Bd. 378

PETER LANG

Frankfurt am Main · Berlin · Bern · Bruxelles · New York · Oxford · Wien

Kingsley Ufuoma Omoyibo

Adolescent Females' Reproductive Health in Nigeria

A Study on the Legislation and Socio-Cultural Impediments to Abortion and against Female Circumcision

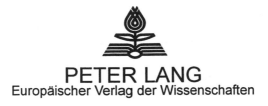

PETER LANG
Europäischer Verlag der Wissenschaften

Die Deutsche Bibliothek - CIP-Einheitsaufnahme

Omoyibo, Kingsley Ufuoma:

Adolescent females' reproductive health in Nigeria : a study on
the legislation and socio-cultural impediments to abortion and
against female circumcision / Kingsley Ufuoma Omoyibo. -
Frankfurt am Main ; Berlin ; Bern ; Bruxelles ; New York ;
Oxford ; Wien : Lang, 2002
    (European university studies ; Ser. 22, Sociology ;
    Vol. 378)
    Zugl.: Berlin, Freie Univ., Diss., 2002
    ISBN 3-631-50284-2

Gedruckt mit Unterstützung des
Deutschen Akademischen Austauschdienstes.

D 188
ISSN 0721-3379
ISBN 3-631-50284-2
US-ISBN 0-8204-6058-3

© Peter Lang GmbH
Europäischer Verlag der Wissenschaften
Frankfurt am Main 2002
All rights reserved.

All parts of this publication are protected by copyright. Any
utilisation outside the strict limits of the copyright law, without
the permission of the publisher, is forbidden and liable to
prosecution. This applies in particular to reproductions,
translations, microfilming, and storage and processing in
electronic retrieval systems.

Printed in Germany 1 2 , 4 5 6 7

www.peterlang.de

Dedicated to all adolescent females' in Nigeria

Acknowledgement

In a work of this nature, its completion would have been impossible without the help and assistance of very consequential individuals and institutions. It is on this note I wish to express my unreserved thanks to my dissertation supervisor, Frau Prof. Dr. Helgard Kramer for her meticulous comments, criticisms and guidance throughout the course of this research work and for making my stay in Germany a memorable one. Madam, you are a real gem. My thanks also go to my second supervisor, Herr Prof. Dr. Johannes Gordesch for his constructive comments and his constant faith in me, from the beginning till the end of this work. Prof. M.A. Onwuejeogwu is also highly acknowledged for his guidance and critical comments on this work during my fieldwork in Nigeria and his academic visit to the Institut für Soziologie, FU-Berlin, in Germany. Sir, I owe you a lot of respect. My thanks also extend to Frau Dr. Ulrike Schultz for her constructive comments on the work.

My un-quantifiable thanks go to my sponsor-The German Academic Exchange Service (DAAD) for the scholarship award without which it would have been difficult for me to have, had the exposure of a developed western blend academic experience at a higher level like the Doctor of Philosophy. To the DAAD, I promise to hold dear your values of excellence.

On records also, are my graduate colleagues at the Institute für Soziologie, FU - Berlin. Worthy of mention is Herr Roger Naegele with whom I established a wonderful friendly relationship both at the academic and social levels. Also, not left out in this appreciation is the authority of University of Benin, Nigeria, my employer for giving me the opportunity through a study leave to actualise the highest point of my academic career. By extension, my special thanks go to all my colleagues in the Sociology department UNIBEN, for their wonderful cooperation during the course of my study.

My invaluable impressions recognizes the roles played the Ogiribo family especially Mark, Late James (RIP), and Daniel for the umpteenth time, you are all more than a brother. I owe much gratitude to all my numerous friends especially, Raymond Koko, Ojo Collins, Aideyan Osaore, Enogie Erhabor, Sievoadje Godwin, Ukpebor Emma, Okoro Kingsley, Iyayi Eromosele, who were always there when it mattered most.

My special thanks goes to my parents Mr. And Mrs. A. Omoyibo, for their initial interest in my academic career, which was not a mistake; and to all my brothers and sisters for their special prayers and understanding during the course of my study.

In the course of this academic sojourning, I came across other nice folks like Inegbedion, Izamojie, Afonoghara, Egbivwie, Sola, Tzanaka Kokalova, Kuczma Magdalena, Alex Ali, Chris Dück, Daniel Tsegai, Tesfaye Baye, Adeniran, W., and Frau Elke Tischer (my Professor's secretary). The members of Association of Nigerian Students, and Urhobo Progress Union (UPU), Germany branch are also acknowledged. Please endeavour to keep the good spirit of association on.

This acknowledgement would be bereft of completion if I fail to recognize a very important segment of persons who made this work a reality, it is in this light, I salute all of my respondents who obliged information, and my research assistants who were always there to make sure the work was done. I thank you all.

Above all, I thank the almighty God for his infinite mercies, providence and guidance to have seen me successfully through this ultimate academic hurdle of my life.

Berlin, im Juli 2002.

List of Tables

Table of Contents

Abstract

One clear indication, of the poor state of reproductive health in Nigeria, has been the failure of well design policies through yawning gap between plans and achievement, that is propelled by lack of efficient implementation. Much more, is the discrimination and exclusion of such policies against adolescents generally, the woman and adolescent females in particular. Since 1960s, researches on reproductive health issues have clearly out focused attention on matters that affect the adolescent female or the girl child like abortion and female circumcision. This has led to a tunnel in vision on the part of government in rendering her stewardship in the forms of providing some focus on legislation through the issuing of regulations, decrees, and public orders as means of population policies that affect the health of the girl child.

The factors that mostly affect the health of the girl child revolve around the biological, social, economic, cultural, religious and environmental. The immediate causes are the low status of women in the society arising from their low education, and low earning power, while bearing the double burden of production and reproduction and are yet not fully or effectively integrated in the development process.

These conditions are the key factors that have led to the rising incidence of adolescent maternal deaths that keep arising from illegal termination of unwanted pregnancies and female circumcision. The government on her part is being constrained to embrace the option of legalization of abortion and legislation against female circumcision because of the strong influence of socio-cultural factors that are deeply rooted in the society.

Sex preference seems to have had serious effects overtime on major population policies as it affects women and adolescents health. There is good evidence that male preference has influenced the treatment and low social status of women in most Nigerian communities, especially among the Urhobo, Okpe, Isoko and Bini ethnic groups.

This research critically evaluates the reproductive health system in Nigeria as it affect the adolescent female and, the legislative and socio-cultural impediments to abortion and against female circumcision. It highlights some of the legislative and socio-cultural loopholes of population policies as it affect reproductive health, and the dangers it has had on women's health and, uphold that improvement in social conditions of the woman or girl child can be attained with improved greater education and development, as well as improved access to qualitative reproductive health services.

The research is qualitative and descriptive in approach with simple and minimal quantitative data infusions to illuminate it where necessary. To do this the study relied on information from adolescent and adult males and females, legislators, orthodox and unorthodox health experts, Women Right Activists and legal practitioners.

The hypotheses on abortion, female circumcision and the stated assumptions on reproductive health were also analysed and evaluated respectively. The mode of data collection was multivariate, through focus group discussions and personal interviews (including case studies) sessions. Other sources included government documents, gazettes, library research, web resources on reproductive health and gender issues.

The research revealed that greater attention be focussed on education of women; awareness and enlightenment campaigns targeted at both religious and community leaders who still enjoy the confidence and respect of the people to help in the mobilization campaign of their congregation and subjects respectively, by emphasizing the dangers of female circumcision and the problem encountered by adolescent females procuring illegal abortion; and the need to re-examine the utility of photos and videos in studying reproductive and sexuality health issues, and documenting the hazardous aspects of female circumcision and illegal abortion, as well as re-orientating the socialization process of all members of society in the direction of gender equality rather than gender preference.

The study findings show no significant advantages of female circumcision beyond the fact that it is a long held traditional practice, and made recommendations on how government should embark on the formulation of effective national legislative policies to ban or outlaw the practice of female circumcision and, also to legislate on the liberalization or legalization of abortion in order to improve the health and sexuality of the girl child. Government should do this without being seen as targeting the cultures or traditions of the people.

1.0.Chapter one: Introduction

1.1. Background of Study

Reproductive health is a state of complete physical, mental and social well - being and not merely the absence of disease and infirmity, in all matters relating to the reproductive system and to its functions and processes.[1] Reproductive health therefore implies that people are able to have a satisfying and safe sex life and that they have the capability to reproduce and freedom to decide if, when and how often to do so. Some of the components of sexual and reproductive rights include, reproductive and sexual health, reproductive decisions making, equality and equity for men and women, and sexual and reproductive security. The consequences of denying these sexual and reproductive rights of women result in high rate of maternal mortality and maternal morbidity due to unsafe abortion, female genital mutilation, and other domestic and sexual violence[2]

Reproductive health care has a central role to play in the prevention of all known consequences in the fight against reproductive health problems. According to universally agreed standard, everyone has the right to comprehensive, good quality reproductive health services that ensures privacy, fully informed and free consent, confidentiality and respect for the client. However, for huge numbers of people these rights mean precious little at present, for they lack access to even the most basic care because of intervening social variables like lack of female education, retrogressive cultural beliefs and practices, lack of female decision making, lack of economic resources and government unwillingness to co-operate. The above issues are very crucial in understanding the plight of the adolescents who constitutes one of the largest categories of human groups in most societies. In fact, one out of every five people in the world is an adolescent. Like many other groups, adolescents all of the world have specific concerns and problems.

---

[1] Document and Resolutions of the International Conference on Population and Development (ICPD), Cairo, 1994 Pp. 43; and Friday E. Okonofua (editorial) on 'Infertility and Reproductive Health in Africa.' *African Journal of Reproductive Health*, 1999, Vol.3 (1), Pp. 7-10; and 'Reproductive Health As a Fundamental Human Right' Unpublished manuscript by Friday E. Okonofua 1994, Pp. 10-14
[2] Friday E. Okonofua 1994, Pp. 10.

The Convention on the Rights of the Child, addresses the human rights of all persons below age 18,and since most people who are considered adolescents are below the age of 19, the children's convention encompasses their human rights.[3] The Programme of Action at the 1994 International Conference on Population and Development (ICPD) and the 1995 Platform for Action at the Forth World Conference on Women (FWCW) provide that reproductive rights embrace certain human rights that are already recognised in national laws, international human rights documents and other consensus documents. The children's convention is one of the key international human rights documents that contain numerous provisions encompassing the reproductive health rights of the adolescents as stated in the ICPD and FWCW programme of actions. Among the hardest fought provisions were 'the guarantees of young peoples rights to confidential information and services for sexual and reproductive health. Ultimately, both conferences included extensive and unprecedented agreements on this issue.' (ICPD 1994, Paragraphs. 7.41, 7.45 to 7.47; FWCW 1995, Paragraphs 83/, 106m, 107e, and g, 108k, 108/, 267, 281e and g); in this context, recognition of adolescents' rights is essential to reduce both the high rates of unwanted teenage pregnancy and large numbers of unsafe abortions in this age group as well as to help them to understand the health issues associated with female circumcision.

However, there remains a significant gap between the provisions contained in the Children's Convention and the reality of adolescent's reproductive health and lives. Many organizations, religious bodies, non-governmental organizations, and women groups and associations have addressed adolescents reproductive health rights issues and have come up with many concluding observations to governments, often stressing the need for government to take steps to ensure these rights. In too many cases, governments and societies have tended either to ignore adolescent's reproductive health issues or to consider them indistinguishable from childhood health concerns. This is observed from the law banning abortion that has made many adolescent females emergency mothers, and the physical pains undergone by many due to female circumcision. In both circumstances, many adolescent females have undergone both physical and emotional trauma without being matured physically and emotionally.

In Nigeria, the situation of female adolescents reproductive health is worsened by the gender phenomenon. In this context, gender refers to the different roles of

---

[3] Convention on the Rights of the Child, article 1 'Opened for Signature.' November 20, 1989. General Assembly Resolution 44/25, U.N.G.A. Order of Resolution, 44th session, supp. No. 49; U.N. Document A/44/49, reprinted in 28 I.L.M. 1448 (entry into force September 2, 1990) (hereinafter Children's Convention). The Provision states that "for purposes of the present convention a child means every human being below the age of 18 years unless, under the law applicable to the child, majority is attained later."

males and females, as determined by the society and culture in which they live in. Society places a higher value on males than females. Consequently, gender roles and norms have a major impact on the reproductive health of young adults especially the females.[4] Also, gender affect expectations regarding the sexual activities of boys and girls, and these differences in expectations create separate standards for males and females in terms of social consequences of reproductive health.

Today, abortion and female circumcision are considered the two most controversial reproductive health issues in population policy debate in Nigeria that affects adolescent females. While abortion is out rightly illegal except to save the life of the woman, it also accounts for the highest cause of maternal mortality in Nigeria. Of the estimated 50,000 maternal deaths every year, approximately 20,000 results from the complications of unsafe and induced abortion. Of those women admitted to hospitals for complications due to abortion, about eighty per cent of them are adolescents.[5] Thus, lack of safe legal abortion services for adolescents jeopardizes their health and lives and undermines their rights to make decisions concerning childbearing as indicated in the Children's Convention that protects the rights to life and health of all children without limitation.

On female circumcision, there is no critical legal and policy measure in place to curb its perpetuation amongst practising ethnic groups. Its prevalence rate range from 15-100 per cent depending on ethnic group; in 1985-1986 the National Association of Nigerian Nurses and Midwives (NANNM) conducted a survey of female genital mutilation practices in the then nineteen states, and in five states an estimated 90 per cent of women underwent some type of genital mutilation. In the state of Kaduna 15 per cent of women were infibulated, 45 per cent were excised and 35 per cent were circumcised. Presently, Nigeria has a total national prevalence of about fifty per cent of women who are circumcised.[6]

More so, abortion and female circumcision tend to be affected by the position of tradition and culture. For instance, tradition and culture tend to compel young women to seek abortions, as there are strong social sanctions against unmarried women with children, and an unmarried pregnant woman.[7] This same tradition is contradictory in condemning abortion as killing and murder on the part of perpetrators. While on the other hand it serves as the social agent that, propel the act itself. On female circumcision, tradition gives meaning to its continuity, such as enhancing fertility, easing childbirth, curbing promiscuity, neatness of the vagina, rite of passage to womanhood etc.

---

[4] USAID 1996, Gender Plan of Action: Bringing Beijing Home. Gender Action, 1(1), Pp. 3
[5] I. F. Adewole 1992, Pp. 115-118.
[6] Efua Dorkenoo 1995, Pp. 107.
[7] B. Suleiman 1996, Pp. 1.

Religious arguments have also been advanced to interfere with legislation on abortion and against female circumcision. While Islam, Christianity and tradition hold that it is against God's commandment to kill; on the other hand, it is clear that female circumcision has no strong basis either in Islam or Christianity, but religion is only interpreted by, chauvinistic leaders to endorse the subjugation of women.[8]

Nigerian society like many other societies in the world does not pretend to the fact that, adolescent sexuality is very sensitive. Furthermore, that most adolescents receive little or no health or sexuality education, and many are completely ignorant of their bodies, reproduction, contraception, diseases prevention to mention a few. They are generally unlikely to use sexual health services that are for adults; and services designed for adolescents are extremely rare. Consequently, most of them are subjected to bodily harm like female circumcision; exposed to unwanted pregnancies and procurement of illegal abortion through getting dangerous clandestine abortions that could result in the contraction of STDs and HIV/AIDS and in most cases, result to serious illnesses, infertility or deaths.

In Nigeria, where abortion and female circumcision are mostly performed by back street traditional midwives and herbalists under unsanitary conditions because of the laws on the restriction of the earlier, and the lack of legislative policy regulating the later, it is important and urgent that almost no where can access to adolescents females reproductive health can be taken for granted as stated in the consensus documents agreed to at the International Conference on Population and Development (ICPD) and the Forth World Conference on Women (FWCW) which explicitly recognise that "everyone has the right to the enjoyment of the highest attainable standard of physical and mental health". This include the right to reproductive health defined in both documents, "…that all individuals have such rights, without qualification as to marital status, age or any other classification" (International Conference of Human Rights, UN-Document 1968. Tehran, Proclamation). In particular, Article 24 of both documents recognises children's right "…to the enjoyment of the highest standard of health and to facilities for the treatment of illness and rehabilitation of health. It also requires states parties to take appropriate measures to develop family planning education services…."[9] At both conferences, adolescent reproductive health was considered as a major human rights issue to which many countries were urged to subscribe and to expand, promote and invigorate. In pursuance of these responsibilities, Nigerian government that was not only participant and a signatory to both documents in concert with non-governmental organizations should act with greater determination to address the reproductive health concerns of adolescents.

---

[8] Efua Dorkenoo 1995, Pp. 39.
[9] Children Convention, Article 24 (f), UN-Document, 1990 A/44/49

1.2. Statement of Research Problem

The World Health Organization (WHO) estimates that one-tenth of the world's population is aged between 15-19 years old, 80 percent of who live in the developing countries. In most societies both North and South, adolescents are more sexually active. In fact, adolescent mothers account for one fifth of all births each year. Nevertheless, adolescent sexuality is still a taboo in many societies.[10]

In the Nigerian population estimate for 1990, this age group constituted about 20 percent of the total population. This age group is large and growing and studies have shown that it is sexually active. Studies in Nigeria also show that the mean age at first intercourse ranges between 15 and 18 years. Also, the 1981/1982 Nigerian fertility survey reported that the age specific rate for 15-19 age group was 173.3 births per 1,000 during the five years preceding the survey, and evidence suggest that abortion is common in this group. More so, contraceptive knowledge and use was found to be very low.[11] One of the problems that have been identified is the 'conspiracy of silence' surrounding sexuality and reproductive health issues, which has led to its denial as a fundamental dimension of the human being. This has led adolescents at the mercy of an uncontrolled distortion of sexuality. Every unwanted pregnancy represents a failure by society to provide women with ways to avoid it. These include, full information about her body, sexuality, reproduction and contraception and also, access to various services necessary to ensure that she can act on that knowledge. The failure of governments to liberalise laws on abortion has compounded the issue, as it had made adolescents to seek clandestine illegal, unsafe and induced abortion. The consequences of which is death, which often go unrecorded.

Today in Nigeria, any estimate given on the prevalent rate of induced abortion amongst adolescents is at best an intelligent guess, because the operators are as diverse as the methods. However, estimates based on hospital records of induced abortion cases that are referred to it due to complications are alarming.[12] The situation is further worsened knowing that most deaths from illegal abortions go unrecorded, because most deaths occur outside the hospitals and accurate reliable records of such deaths are rarely maintained in private hospitals.

This high estimates of illegal, induced and unsafe abortion is worsened further by the serious health, social, cultural and psychological consequences of unwanted pregnancies and abortions. In addition, the issue of legalizing or liberalizing the existing abortion laws has been saddled by controversies and conflicts. This

---

[10] Gloria Vincent-Osaghae, 'Improving Adolescent Reproductive Health and the Role of Sexuality Education' *Journal For Women's Health Forum,* 1997, Vol.2 (2), Pp. 5

[11] Gloria Vincent-Osaghae 1997, Pp. 5.

[12] J. B. Akingba, et al. 1971, / Pp. 126, O. Adetoro, 1980, Pp. 102-105 / J. A. Unuigbe, et al. 1988, Pp. 435-439.

conflict and controversy emanate from the perception of the adult Nigerian population, a minority of whom may, not have suffered directly or indirectly from the consequences of clandestine and unsafe abortions. More importantly, these perceptions are to a large extent influenced by their cultural, religious and moral inclination.

In the same vein, the issue of female circumcision otherwise known as female genital mutilation (FGM)- a devastating ancient cultural practice with its attendant medical, health, socio-psychological and physical consequences is a violation of not only the information on the woman's control of her body, but also, an abuse of the sexual and reproductive health rights of the adolescent female.

The sexual and reproductive health of adolescent females in Nigeria in respect of abortion and female circumcision is compounded by a host of cultural, legal and economic factors that put women at lower social status and special risks. In many Nigerian societies girls face discriminations from birth onward. Typically, they have less access to education, information and skills training than boys, which handicap them for life. As adults they have limited opportunity often with little or no rights, and also, limited access to health care services. This low social status of women make them socially vulnerable to all forms of discriminatory forces which limit their opportunities to be informed about the functioning of their bodies, sexuality and health, and cripple their autonomy and power to protect themselves. In fact, in many of the multiplicity of the Nigerian cultures, it is considered indecent for a woman to take the initiative in sexual encounters. Thus, they are inhibited from seeking out information on such matters that could improve their sexual and reproductive health.

In all of these, a general omission in the studies on abortion and female circumcision in Nigeria, are the views of adolescent females and the poor who account for a higher percentage of the deaths or physical and emotional damage resulting from their perpetuation either illegally or by back street midwives, non-health providers, untrained orthodox heath providers etc. Attempts to fill the gaps in knowledge about the host of issues surrounding adolescent females reproductive and sexual health behaviour by focussing on original researches published in a review of recent researches since 1990 note that "…obtaining current and complete statistics on adolescent females reproductive health behaviour is problematic because the data came from surveys designed for other purposes, such as the National Survey of Family Growth (NSFG), the National Survey of Adolescent Males (NSAM), and the Youth Risk Behaviour Study (YRBS). All of these sources have limitations that make data analysis difficult. Consequently, adolescent females are more likely to suffer from the restrictive law on abortion and the non existent legislative policy against female circumcision, as well as her poor accessibility and availability to orthodox health services."[13]

Invariably, in the wake of the twenty-first century and the concern of the Nigerian government on the explosive growth in population, increase in the number of maternal mortality resulting from unhealthy reproductive and sexual health issues, global attention on the reproductive rights of women, reduced influence of religious institutions on women's issue because of the internal conflicts between congregation members on what the position of religion should be in this respect, and the wave of liberalized reforms going on at the global level etc, all of these lay credence for the need to examine adolescent females reproductive health in the light of legislations on abortion and against female circumcision in Nigeria.

1.3 The Scope of the Study

This dissertation had as its scope the understanding of the issues of abortion, and female circumcision in the context of the socio-cultural, political and economic life patterns of the people of Sapele, and Ethiope-East local government areas respectively of Delta state, in Nigeria. It also, focussed and emphasized on the adolescent female population and other related reproductive and sexual health behaviours such as STDs, HIV/AIDS infections.

The scope as well entailed understanding the roles of the people's culture and religion as an impediment to legislation on abortion and against female circumcision. The issue of reproductive health rights of the adolescent female and the role of the woman in these complicities was dealt with, as well as the examination of the role of the state in the raging controversy.

1.4 Aims and Objectives

This dissertation was carried out with the following aims and objectives in mind:

• To examine the general laws and practices relating to abortion and female circumcision in Nigeria.

• To ascertain the socio-cultural factors militating against the legislations on abortion and encouraging female circumcision.

• To establish the perception and attitudes of adolescents to the laws, social and cultural dictates restricting their access to abortion and impeding their resistance to female circumcision.

• To ascertain the level of awareness among adolescents of these laws, cultural and medical views on abortion and female circumcision.

---

[13] Adetoun Ilumoka 1991, Pp. 122.

- To establish their knowledge, attitude and practice (KAP) of contraception to control unwanted pregnancies and other reproductive health problems that affects them.

- To propound the positions of adolescents on liberalization of abortion, and legislation against female circumcision.

1.5 Research Hypotheses on Abortion and Female Circumcision

1.5.1 Hypotheses on Abortion

This research has as its hypotheses on abortion the following:

- That adolescent females engage in the use of illegal abortion to terminate unwanted pregnancies

- That adolescent female's, rely on the use of ineffective contraceptives to prevent and induce unwanted pregnancies

- That adolescents have restricted access to safe contraception

- That many adolescents are unaware of the abortion law

- That adolescents advocate the liberalization or legalization of abortion in Nigeria

1.5.2. Hypotheses on Female Circumcision

1.5.2.a. Cultural Hypotheses on Female Circumcision

- That female circumcision enhances women fertility.

- That female circumcision reduces sexual promiscuity on the part of women.

- That female circumcision is a male dictated or controlled aspect of the culture of the practicing areas (for instance, amongst the Urhobo and Okpe speaking ethnic groups, women cannot take political position unless they are excised)

- That there is no relationship between female circumcision and the survival of the child during birth.

1.5.2.b. Medical Hypotheses on Female Circumcision

- That circumcised females are easily prone to HIV/AIDS infections.

- That female circumcision is carried out mostly by traditional midwives and native doctors.

1.5.2.c. Legislative Hypotheses on Female Circumcision

- That adolescent female's are subjected to the act of circumcision against their consent.

- That adolescents advocate a legislative policy to ban the practice of female circumcision.

1.5.3 General Assumptions on Reproductive Health

• That to promote compulsory and free primary and secondary education for all adolescents irrespective of gender with an incorporated program or curriculum on sex education would help in raising the awareness of adolescent females in particular, and women in general on the issue of reproductive and sex issue.

• That the parental factor is very crucial in the socialization process of the child, particularly, at the stage of the adolescent sexual development. That the better the parents play their roles at this period the lesser the number of adolescents that would be victims of reproductive and sexual health hazards.

• That the recognition and incorporation of traditional, community and religious leaders in the mobilization process on the reproductive health rights of the adolescents particularly the females, would help in a much faster way in the dissemination of information about reproductive health and sexual issues.

• That if the socio-economic status of women is enhanced, and poverty amongst them ameliorated to a large extent, this would create an economic, as well as social independence that would help them to take decisions that affects their bodies without much dictates from a society and culture that is gender bias in favour of the male child.

• That if government honours all international conventions signed as it applies to reproductive and sexual health matters of the adolescents in general and the females in particular, most of the discriminations in these respect would be tremendously reduced.

1.6 Justification of the Study

This study is justified on the basis of the following reasons:

First, the growing population in the midst of economic recession in the nascent democratic governance in Nigeria has adversely affected the standard of living of the people. Thus, the average family can barely feed itself and therefore, further pressure from unwanted pregnancies and babies would pose a threat to the individual, family and society.

Second, the economic recession now makes it difficult or impossible for most Orphanage homes and hospitals in Nigeria to cater for their wards nor take in additional abandoned babies; and with no funds coming from government(s), organizations and philanthropists, and the cost of baby milk astronomically high and beyond the reach of many mothers and families; needless to talk of Orphanages, there is therefore the need to curb unwanted pregnancies.

Third, at the moment, the present draft constitution of Nigeria is inadequate in terms of concrete ideas on reproductive and sexual matters as it affects the woman; and debates abound on the draft constitution and government policies on women reproductive rights. It becomes imperative and highly important to contribute and make suggestions based on scientific findings on providing solution towards the control of unwanted pregnancies and the issue of female circumcision- otherwise known as female genital mutilation.

Finally, the Beijing conference of 1995 highlighted some of the problems associated with women; prominent among such include, reproductive rights of the woman, particularly with respect to the legalization or liberalization of abortion globally, and abrogation of all forms of traditions that endorses female genital mutilation (FGM)[14] that has rendered most women physically incapacitated for life, while majority of others had lost their lives during child birth because of the serious tear of the vagina and subsequent loss of blood. Some others have been victims of HIV/AIDS infections in the process of group circumcision operation. Somehow, it has financial burdened on the government.

For these reasons this research stand out as a significant basis for further researches on the fundamental reproductive health rights of adolescent females in particular and women in general.

1.7 Problem with the Study

Major problems, was encountered by this researcher in the process of gathering data. These problems constituted the limitations of the research.

First, there are very few books written on female reproductive health in Nigeria. Worse still, very little has been focussed on adolescent reproductive health. This made this researcher to rely more on general works and reports from the United Nation agencies like; the World Health Organization (WHO), United Nations Children Fund (UNICEF); and on conference reports like, the International Conference on Population and Development (ICPD), Forth World Conference on Women (FWCW); children convention articles, International Conference on Human Rights (ICHR) articles; as well as government gazettes and reports, newspapers and magazines, opinions of individuals etc. to make up the literatures for this work.

Second, the establishment of contacts with respondents as shown in the methodology constituted a serious problem initially. This problem was later surmounted through other familiar contact persons on the basis of trust and confidentiality.

More so, the difficulty on the part of respondents (especially the female) in the various categories to oblige information willingly on the topic of research- abortion and female circumcision, underscored the myths and taboo's surrounding sex related issues in many Nigerian cultures. The cultural

---

[14] Centre for Reproductive law and Policy (CRPL)"Women of the World: Laws and Policies Affecting their Reproductive Lives- Anglophone Africa; and the Open Forum on Reproductive Health and Rights. Women Behind Bars: Chile's Abortion Laws- A Human Rights Analysis. CRPL 1998. 'Supra note' 33 at 172."

backgrounds of the Urhobo, Okpe, Isoko, Ika, Itsekiri and Bini speaking participants accounted for the uncomfortable and shy nature of girls and women in discussing sex related issues either in the presence of males or in the presence of unfamiliar persons. But at such instances my female research assistant intervened in probing into issues or questions that are considered cultural taboos for men to venture into while discussing with women. More so, with consistent education, assurances, explanations, and conviction on the part of the researcher and his trained assistants through the process of participant learning and action (PLA) method respondents and participants got over this mythical conception and obliged information. All of these were time, resource and energy consuming.

Third, as a corollary to the above, most orthodox health providers in both public and private health establishments rejected the idea of been video-recorded. They preferred to talk off records because of what they termed the 'sensitivity of the issues and the laws of the state', as well as the professional ethical requirement in trained medical practice. This underlined the effects of the law on the restriction of abortion and the socio-cultural impact on the issues of both abortion and female circumcision. While on the part of trado-medical or unorthodox health providers, most of them reacted initially to the issue with measures of scepticism, particularly as they saw themselves as been in strict competition with the orthodox medical providers. In spite of these obvious frustrations, their responses were quite frank and revealing.

Noteworthy, is the fact, that public health institutions have no proper documentary records of cases of abortion and female circumcision victims. This was particularly frustrating, as all information in this direction was very sketchy, unreliable and haphazard. Thus efforts made to provide data on cases relating to the research focus over the last 5 and 10 years was not successful. This is as a result of the illegality in perpetuating abortion on the one hand, and the non-acceptance of orthodox health officials to claims of engaging in female circumcision.

Forth, it was also not easy to track down legislators at both the federal and state levels because of their busy schedule, to speak on these issues that is considered of great significant value on my first fieldwork trip. A number of appointments were slated with some of them well ahead of time to ensure that the discussion of the issue went right. With an opportunity given for a second fieldwork trip, this task was accomplished. It should be noted that it took time and series of slated appointments before some of them were reached to speak out on the issues. More so, they all opted to speak off the records because of what they termed an issue of very sensitive cultural implication.

Fifth, the financial involvement in terms of training my research assistants, transportation to cover the area of research, as well as to provide gifts in the form of condoms, and the entertainments of respondents during focussed group and interview sessions was enormous.

Sixth, was the problem that arose from the researchers emotional attachment to the focus of the topic of research; it was initially difficult for this researcher to detach 'self' completely from the issues, particularly during the focus group and the interview sessions. This situation almost replayed itself during the analysis. But with a cautionary reminder of the detachment of 'self from emotional involvement in scientific research'; this researcher was able to manage this effectively to produce an objective dissertation.[15]

Above all, this research was able to integrate the interests of the study population and other concerned interests for a greater practical relevance of the study, which in turn helps to project the image of humane and reliable research.[16]

1.8 Clarification of Research Concepts

1.8.1 Adolescents

Adolescent's has been described by social commentators towards the end of the nineteenth century, as the period of growth between childhood and adulthood.[17] However, in Kett, J. work *'Rite of Passage'* and Hall, Stanley's *'Adolescence.'* They argued 'that adolescence is an even more recent cultural intervention than childhood'. Thus the term adolescent is synonymous with the term 'teenagers'. It is therefore, described as both a period of storm and stress, and also a possibility and promise. Furthermore, Hall Stanley pointed out that teenagers should be given a chance to experiment with and explore various roles available to them before being pushed into the adult world.[18]

The adolescent's stage of growth is likened to other birth cohort that are affected, by their group members (adolescent sub-culture) with whom they interact, and the social and cultural conditions to which they are exposed.[19] Eric, Erikson noted in his book on *'Childhood and Society'* that at this stage of trying to attain maturation, Adolescents are faced with the identity versus role confusion. He defined 'identity as an attempt at understanding who one is and where one is going? In effect, identity is built on a sense of continuity about ones past, present and future. This period is described by Sigmund Freud in his work, *'The Ego and the Id' in 1947*, as one of the most delicate in the development of personality, as adolescents who are unable to develop an identity experience role confusion.[20]

The term adolescence applies to the emotional and behavioural states supposedly associated with becoming adult; the phase in the life circle before the physical

---

[15] G.O. Yomere and Barnabas A. Agbonifo 1999, Pp. 170.
[16] Klaus-Dieter Beißwenger, et. al. 1993, Pp. 76.
[17] Craig Calhoun, et al. 1994, Pp. 140.
[18] Craig Calhoun, et al. 1994, Pp. 141.
[19] Matilda W. Riley 1987, 1987, Pp. 1-2.
[20] Craig Calhoun, et al. 1994, Pp. 110-114.

changes associated with puberty are socially recognized, or the transition in status from childhood to adulthood.[21]

The age at which children become adolescents is currently a source of controversy, as it is now a determination of a number of factors depending on race, ethnic background, religion, social class and other characteristics.[22] In fact, Neugarten, B.L. and Neugarten, D.A. (1987) pointed out that, there are signs that the age at which children become adolescents is slowly creeping downwards-from fifteen or sixteen to only eleven or twelve.[23] Typically, in modern industrial societies, young people are sexually matured well before society acknowledges them as adults in other respects; and, because of education and training, they remain dependent on parents and guardians.[24]

However, in many traditional societies like the Urhobo, Okpe, Bini and Itsekiri speaking peoples of Nigeria, adolescents are those who are between the ages of twelve and twenty-one. While in the statutory code of the land, adolescents are categorised as people between the ages of thirteen and nineteen. This categorisation is applied in the court of law in defining who is a criminal? At the on set of adolescence, sexual maturation and cultural norms combine to produce a new differentiation of behaviour and experience. At this point, sexual satisfaction is at the heart of contemporary adolescents ideas of having fun for both male and female.[25]

For this reason, I adopt the World Health Organization (WHO) definition of adolescents. This is because of its universal standard of application. The WHO defines adolescents as "persons in the 10-19 years age group. While youths as the 15-24 years age group, and young people as a combination of these two overlapping groups covering the range 10-24 years."[26]

1.8.2 Socio-Cultural Factors

These are elements that are embedded in both society and culture that tend to regulate the behavioural patterns of the individual, and group of people in the social system. The contents of this socio-cultural factors include, language, knowledge, signs and symbols, values, norms, artefacts-the physical objects that

---

[21] Gordon Marshall 1998, Pp. 7.

[22] Craig Calhoun, et al. 1994, Pp. 142.

[23] Bernice L. Neugarten and Dail A. Neugarten, 1987, Pp. 29-33.

[24] Gordon Marshall 1998, Pp. 7.

[25] Stephen Heath 1982, Pp. 4-7.

[26] United Nations Population Fund, Technical and Policy Division Draft Report, 'The Sexual and Reproductive Health of Adolescents 2, April, 1998.' Hereinafter Sexual and Reproductive Health of Adolescents; and 'The Health of Youth: Fact for Action, Youth and Nutrition Document A/42/Technical Discussion/2, Geneva: W.H.O., 1989a.'

the people make; as well as the social structure, institutions, sub-systems, folktales, folklores, mores, customs, traditions etc.[27]

Although, the contents of socio-cultural factors varies from place to place, it is also, known that all human societies and cultures have the same basic elements, and people use these as the socio-cultural 'tool kits' both to maintain and to change their ways of life.[28]

1.8.3 Legislation

Legislation simply refers to the laws that are made by a legal authority that exist in a place or defined territory at any particular point in time.[29] Therefore, legislations are different from norms because "they are formalized or codified laws, which are rules enacted by a political body and enforced by the power of the state. Thus, legislations are enforced by the police, the military or by other specialized organizations."[30] However, there are known cases where legislations help to formalize folkways, folklores, mores or norms. In general, legislations that are most difficult to enforce are those that are not grounded in folkways or mores. For example, laws against gambling or drinking before age twenty-one.

1.8.4 Abortion and Contraception

These terms has been defined from multi-disciplinary perspectives. These include, medical, social, economic, cultural, religious and psychological perspectives. Nevertheless, they all convey similar meanings and understanding. This research however, adopts a simple and unambiguous definition for the purpose of easy comprehension and the attainment of its spelt out aims and objectives.

Davis, et al (1985), defines abortion "as the expulsion of the product of conception from the uterus prior to the stages of viability (about 24 to 28 weeks gestation). While, the prevention of pregnancy in sexual activity is referred to as contraception or birth control". Therefore, while contraception is the prevention of pregnancy, abortion on the other hand, is the termination of pregnancy before the foetus is matured enough to survive outside the uterus.[31]

Abortion, fall into two categories, - spontaneous and induced. Spontaneous abortion, occur naturally in the form of miscarriages. While induced abortions, are those caused to terminate, pregnancy. This can be in the form of dilation and curettage (D and C), through the dilation of the cervix. On the other hand contraception method involve natural contraceptive means in the form of fertility awareness, or mechanical contraceptives (condoms, diaphragms, IUDs, etc);

---

[27] Ikechukwu Enwemnwa 1995, Pp. 2, and Craig Calhoun, et al. 1994, Pp. 62, 97-99

[28] Ann Swindler 1986, Pp. 273.

[29] Hawkins 1995, Pp. 232.

[30] Craig Calhoun, et al. 1994, Pp. 58.

[31] Bowman O. Davis, et al. 1985, Pp. 558.

14

chemical contraceptives (killing sperm crèmes, oral pills etc); surgical contraception method (vasectomy, tubal litigation etc.)

1.8.5 Female Circumcision

This term has been described in many ways. They include, operation, excision, maiming, wounding, cutting, damaging, defacing and mutilation etc. of the female genitalia. But for the purpose of this research study, the definition of the World Health Organization (WHO) is adopted because of its universal standard and acceptance.

The WHO defines female circumcision as "all procedures involving partial or total removal of the female external genitalia or other injuries to the female genital organs whether for cultural or other non-therapeutic reasons."[32] The WHO further expanded the definition by classifying four types of female circumcision, which is a reflection of minor to very complicated procedures of the practice. These are as follows:

Type 1

This is the excision of the prepuce, with or without excision of part or all of the, clitoris. This procedure, also include ritualistic circumcision, sunna, and clitoridectomy.

Type 2

This is the excision of the clitoris with partial or total excision of the labia minora.

Type 3

This is the excision of part or all of the external genitalia and stitching or narrowing of the vagina opening (infibulation). This procedure includes, the pharaonic circumcision and Somalian circumcision.

Type 4

These are the category termed unclassified. They include, pricking, piercing, or incising of the clitoris and or the labia; stretching of the clitoris and or labia; cauterisation by burning of the clitoris and surrounding tissue; scrapping of tissues surrounding the vagina orifice (angurya cuts) or cutting of the vagina (gishiri cuts); introduction of corrosive substances or herbs into the vagina to cause bleeding or for the purpose of tightening or narrowing it; and any other procedure which fall under the definition of female circumcision.[33]

---

[32] 'Female Genital Mutilation, report of W.H.O. Technical Working Group, July 17-19, 1995, Pp. 9, in Geneva Switzerland; and Unpublished Document of WHO/FRH/WHD/96:10, Geneva, 1996

[33] World Health Organization 1995, Pp. 9.

The practice of female circumcision that is regarded as a custom dates back to at least 2,000 years.[34] It is instructive to note that until the 1950's female circumcision was performed in England and the United States of America as a common treatment for lesbianism, masturbation, hysteria, epilepsy and other so called female deviances. In fact, as far back as 1866, an American medical journal discussed the work of a British physician, Dr. Isaac Brown Baker, who claimed success in treating epilepsy, and other nervous disorders in female patients by excising the clitoris.[35]

Today, the complications associated, with this practice has made it a global conscious public health issue that requires legislation to curb its continuous practice. Some of the immediate physical problems ranges from intense pains and or haemorrhage, shock, anaemia, wound infection, especially tetanus, damage to adjoining organs and urine retention. While the long term complications include, painful or blocked menses, recurrent urinary track infections (UTI), abscesses, dermoid cysts and keloid scars, obstructed labour, infertility, psychosomatic illnesses, risk of the contraction of HIV which can further result in the contraction of AIDS; delay in sexual arousal or impairment of orgasm and painful intercourse etc: These motley of problems make female circumcision one of the greatest un-measurable reproductive and sexual health horrors.[36] However, of relevance is the point, mentioned by Fran Hosken (1993)) that, "the highest maternal and infant mortality rates are in female circumcision practicing regions of the world."[37]

1.8.6. Orthodox and Unorthodox Health Experts

The term orthodox health experts was used in this study to define, individuals who underwent the conventional western form of medical and paramedical training in recognized formal institutions that are accredited for the award of certificates in the various aspects of medical specialization, for instance, nurses, pharmacists, health technologist, laboratory technologists, medical doctors etc. On the other hand, unorthodox health experts are those who did not go through the conventional process of western medical training, but went through informal traditional process of apprenticeship in the learning of trado-medicine, for example, native or traditional doctors, herbalists, traditional midwives, medium, etc. many of whom are issued certificate of practice by the state or federal ministry of health for the purpose of certification and records. The idea is to control the practice from infiltrators of all sorts.

---

[34] W.G. Rathmann 1959, Pp. 115.
[35] John Duffy 1989, Pp. 1-4.
[36] Awake 1999, Pp. 7.
[37] Fran P. Hosken 1993, Pp. 37.

2.0. Chapter two

2.1. Abortion and Contraception: A Cross-National Trend

Studies on abortion and contraception abound in both developing and developed societies. Generally, the emphasis in these studies highlights the medical consequences of abortion and the need to legalize abortion. Moreover, a few cross-national studies examine the abortion situation in countries with restrictive and liberal or legalized abortion laws using hospital records and data.

In Nigeria, studies have shown that abortion constitutes a substantial proportion of gynaecological and obstetric admissions in hospitals.[38] These data show that higher proportions of these cases that reach the hospitals with serious complications are adolescents.[39] Other studies in the past two decades support earlier studies that more than 60 percent of these hospital cases were adolescents and unmarried women.[40]

This Nigerian pattern differs from that of other African, Asian, Latin American and South American women. Studies have established that the typical abortion patient is a 15-16 years old unmarried school girl with no previous pregnancies.[41] Gatara and Mariuki (1985) showed using the health statistics of Lesotho government that 45 percent of abortions were performed for people 15-24 years.[42]

A more differential pattern is shown in the study in countries with liberalized or legalized abortion laws. Researches on Jamalpur, Bangladesh showed that the death case ratio is lower among women below 25 years than for older women.[43] Similarly, in a report released in Colombia in 1992, it revealed a vital statistics of 1982, which showed that 20 percent of abortions to Colombian women were to women 15-20 years. It further revealed that 73 percent of all Colombian women seeking abortion were married. Prada, et al. (1989) study of Bogota, Colombia further supports the data from vital statistics of 1987. This study carried out by Prada at "The Institute Materno-Infantile" with their in-house database showed that from 1980-1986, 3,000 women were attended to at the clinic with abortion complications. 20 percent of these women were under 20 years. Since 1987, approximately 2,000 abortions have been seen and 23 percent were under 20 years.[44]

---

[38] E. A. Omu, et al. 1981, Pp. 495-499; and Akingba, et al. 1971, Pp. 126
[39] J. A. Unuigbe, et al. 1988, Pp. 435-439, and E. A. Omu, et al. 1981, Pp. 495-499.
[40] J. Akingba, et al. 1969, Pp. 1-4, / J. B. Akingba 1971, Pp. 126, / and S. E. Okojie 1976, Pp. 517
[41] Paul, 1993, Pp. 745.
[42] H. T. Gatara and P. W. Mariuki 1985, Pp. 41.
[43] S. Khan, et al. 1991, Pp. 1184.
[44] E. Prada, et al. 1989, Pp. 33-43.

There is also sufficient data to highlight that induced abortion among adolescent girls are extra-ordinarily high in Nigeria, compared with other developed countries like the United Kingdom, Denmark and Sweden. These, has been highlighted in a number of studies.[45] For example, Society of Gynaecology and Obstetrics of Nigeria (SOGON) in a memorandum addressed to the Federal Government in 1974 urged her to reform the existing laws on abortion in Nigeria. This attempt yielded no result. Again, in 1991 further pressure was put on the government, which made the then Federal Minister of Health, Professor Ransome Kuti to point out to the nation the importance of legalizing abortion. Since then there has been an upsurge in enlightenment activities among individuals and liberal groups such as Women In Nigeria (WIN) on the benefits to the individual and the country if abortion is legalized.

Although, most people argue that legalizing abortion will increase promiscuity and sexual activity among teenagers, studies from countries with liberalized abortion laws do not portray such pattern. Rather, studies on Singapore experience which examined the events leading to the liberalization of abortion laws, the women's changing attitudes towards abortion, methods of abortion and the effects of legalized abortion on the incidence of illegal abortion, made a number of findings. More importantly, three quarters of single women who had abortions were above 20 years of age, while the number of teenage abortions however, has not proportionately increased, remaining relatively stable at around eight to nine per cent of all abortions and women of higher social class (measured by education) were less likely to continue with an unplanned or unwanted pregnancy.[46] Also, Chen's study using national surveys showed that there are, rising levels of conventional contraceptive practice among the population even when abortion rates were increasing.

Similar study showed that in developing society such as Tunisia, liberalizing abortion laws improves contraception and does not lead to excessive use or abuse of abortion, nor does it burden hospital services.[47] This pattern supports evidences from developed or industrialized countries such as United States,[48] Britain or U.K.,[49] and Japan[50] that "Contraceptive practice can improve in the presence of liberal abortion legislation" and invariably reduce the incidence rate of unwanted teenage pregnancies and illegal abortion practices. However, further studies noted that the actual incidence rates of legal abortions fall below those found in countries with similar liberalized abortion laws but resemble more

---

[45] J. Akingba 1971, Pp. 126 and Society of Gynaecology and Obstetrics of Nigeria (SOGON) report, 1974, Pp. 5-8.
[46] P. Chen, et al. 1982, Pp. 38-42.
[47] Nazer 1980, Pp. 488-492.
[48] Christopher Tietze and Sarah Lewit 1972, Pp. 79-119.
[49] P. Diggory 1970, Pp. 231.
[50] Maramatsu, 1960, Pp. 153

closely those allowing abortion only on socio-medical grounds.[51] Also, liberalization of abortion laws in Tunisia has permitted abortions to be performed openly and safely.

However, studies from countries with restrictive laws shows, that incidence of illegal abortions are high and use of safe contraception is low among women of reproductive age 15-49 years. But it is particularly higher in teenage girls or adolescents below 21years of age.[52]

In substantiating the above claim, Francisco Javier Serna Alvarado, the president of the Commission for Health and Social Services in Mexico city, stated in 1999 "that nearly 500,000 abortions are performed in Mexico every year, and that a large percentage of these end the mother's life, and many others result in serious complications that require medical attention and even hospitalisation". He noted further, "that clandestine abortion is the third highest cause of maternal death in Mexico, and that in some cases, crude abortion techniques are employed - introducing sharp pointed objects, taking abortive medication of herbal teas and even throwing oneself down the stairs; the consequences of which includes serious haemorrhages, perforation of the uterus, sterility, infections, and loss of the womb."[53]

Kakembo, (1999), painting a gory picture of the East Africa abortion experience, stated that "about 80,000 mother's die during abortion, and another 20 million carry out unsafe abortions in the world annually and majority of the unsafe abortions are in developing countries." He noted further that, "one in every 10 pregnancies is terminated through unsafe abortion." He attributed the reasons for abortion as due, to several society values, cultural, political and economic factors that discriminates against mothers. He also, stated that teenage pregnancies out of wedlock are abhorred in most cultures. This is because the family from where the pregnant girl hails loses social status; and that single women in political circles are hounded when they get pregnant without a known spouse; consequently, they engage in abortion under any guise.[54]

A review of the United Nations Sub-regions statistics shows that, East Africa with 36 unsafe abortions in every 1,000 women aged between 15-49 has the highest unsafe abortion rate in the world.[55] It also, stated further that this figure is in comparison with other countries in Central Africa with 28 mothers dying per 1,000. However, the World Health Organization (WHO) document titled,

---

[51] P. Chen, et al. 1982, Pp. 38-44.
[52] O. O. Adetoro 1986, Pp. 103; Awake 1999, Pp. 14; P. E. Bailey, et al. 1988, Pp. 27-41, K. Chaturachinda, et al. 1981, Pp.259; E. A. Omu, et al. 1981, Pp. 498; J. A. Unuigbe 1988, Pp. 435-439.
[53] Originally reported in the El-Universal newspaper from which an extract was published in the Awake Christian Magazine edition of May 22, 1999; Pg. 29
[54] Titus Kakembo 1999, Pp. 1.
[55] The Monitor, 1999, Pp. 1.

"Abortion: Global and Regional Estimates of Incidence and Mortality from Unsafe Abortion", shows that abortion occurs highest in areas where it is illegal especially in East Africa.

In underscoring the need to achieve legal and social reform in the laws relating to abortion and contraception in most countries, which constitutes an important area of reproductive health, Nunes and Delph (1997) pointed out that, "the legalization of abortion does not lead to an increase in abortion rates... some of the countries with the lowest abortion rates have the most liberal abortion laws."[56] They also explained in the process that, through liberalization of abortion, not only would maternal mortality and morbidity will be reduced, but that health care costs of abortions and their sequel would also decline and that recourse to abortion itself would be drastically minimized. They therefore noted, in this regards that the, United Nation Population Fund (UNFPA) activities should be extended to the following; provision of safe abortion services, Pre and Post-abortion counselling including family planning, early diagnosis and management of complications or the consequences of unsafe abortion; and the training and advocacy for legal reforms. To them this has become necessary because legislation banning abortions does not prevent women from terminating pregnancies but causes them to resort to illegal and unsafe abortions especially from the Guyanese women experience.

2.2. Abortion and Contraception within the Framework of Pro and Anti Socio-Cultural and Legal Politics

Since man learned how to reproduce, there has been an eternal question of unwanted reproduction, ancient societies performed infanticide by means as primitive as leaving children on the sides of the mountains. With the advent of technology, slowly and surely, man has developed more efficient ways of sparing unwanted children from unworthy parents to the point past infanticides. Abortion, therefore, becomes a process in which a pregnant mother has undesired foetus removed from her body, ceasing the development of potential life into an actual child and sparing the potential child the indignity of coming into life and being killed.[57]

In 1955, the anthropologist George Devereux, in his work *"A Typological Study of Abortion in 350 Primitive, Ancient and Pre-Industrial Societies"* in therapeutic abortion, demonstrated that abortion has been practiced in almost all existing human communities from the earliest time, and that the patterns of abortion use, in hundred of societies around the world since before recorded history, have been strikingly similar. According to him, women faced with

---

[56] F. E. Nunes and Y. M. Delph 1997, Pp. 66.
[57] Ashr Aiwase, May Andi, Matt Salazar and Tracy Tarkington, 'Pro-Choice, Pro-Life methods and alternatives: Supreme Court rulings on abortion, 1973-1994' (Sociology 308c Peace and Conflict) Spring Semester, 1998

unwanted pregnancies turned to abortion regardless of religious and legal sanctions and often at considerable risk. Hence, Chase Nan, in his book "Abortion: A Long History Can't Be Stopped" stated that, 'since abortion is used to deal with upheavals in personal, family and community life, it has been called a fundamental aspect of human behaviour'

In the same vein, primitive tribal societies, practiced abortions through inducement by using poisonous herbs, sharp sticks, or by share pressure on the abdomen until virginal bleeding occurred.[58] In fact, the ancient Chinese and Egyptians had their methods and recipes to cause abortion, while the Greek and Roman civilizations considered abortion an integral part of maintaining a stable population. They also had various poisons administered in various ways, including through tampons. Even renowned ancient philosophers like Socrates, Plato and Aristotle were all known to have suggested abortion.[59] Even Hippocrates who spoke against abortion because he feared injury to the woman, recommended it on occasion by prescribing violent exercises. It was learned that the Roman morality placed no social stigma on abortion.

Globally, abortion is an issue that burns deep lines in nations, amongst people who vehemently view the act as either murder or mercy. In 1973 abortion was legalized in the United States after years of " back-alley doctors" performed the practice with instruments as crude as even a coat hanger, this decision allowed abortion clinics to give rise, offering a safe and healthy environment for individuals and couples to turn in a time of need. The debate, support an unborn infant's right to life and those who support an unwilling mother's right to choose to terminate her own pregnancy.[60]

The controversy raging on 'abortion and contraception' came into prominence as the general main thrust of various governments development policies to improve the health and welfare of their population through various activities including, maternal and child health, and family planning. The intention was for it to serve as both an influence on fertility control and population growth. While this situation met with not much of resistance in developed countries, the reverse is the case in Africa.

Today, this very sentimental issue has taken a global trend of debate, as to 'what the meaning of life is?' In fact, the issue of abortion has been seen as one of the most explosive discussions in most recent times, igniting raging debates in political, medical, social, demographic and theological fields.[61] In the United States, 'Pro- lifers'- otherwise known as anti-abortion advocates marched for the rights of the unborn. While the 'Pro- choice' camp - otherwise known as pro-

---

[58] Henry P. David 1981, Pp. 1
[59] Wendells Watters 1976, Pp. 52.
[60] Ibid
[61] Awake, 1993, Pp. 3.

abortion advocates stand on the grounds of freedom and a woman's rights to decide. The later group are also referred to as the advocates of the reproductive rights of the woman. Crusaders battle freedom fighters in elections, in courts rooms, in churches, even in the streets.

Seager, et al (1997), pointed out that, "governments are key players in the reproductive lives of women worldwide. He stated further that to the extent that governments may provide access to reproductive health and information services, their involvement in population issues can be benign; and that when the controls of women's fertility becomes construed as a matter of National and International policy, there is cause for concern. He explained further that, a powerful network of rich world donors and government provides international population assistance. With this encouragement, an increasing number of governments in poor countries had adopted interventionist population policies. For the sake of population control, many pay little regard to women's rights or their health."[62]

Reacting to the above situation from a 'socio-cultural African perspective', Lynn, Thomas in a publication titled *'Imperial Concerns to Women Affairs: State Effort to Regulate Clitoridectomy and Eradicate Abortion in Meru, Kenya* stated, that abortion is seen as reprehensible by the people because from his interview, with most members of the community, the United Nations documents which puts Kenya in the danger of legalized abortion, contains a misleading language. In his view, reproductive health, which is a crucial term in the document, is defined by the World Health Organization (WHO) "as including access to methods of fertility regulations- which in turn includes, interruption of unwanted pregnancies, and abortion on demand." Furthermore, he pointed out that, "the people see it as shameful that rich Western countries and International Organizations are putting pressures on Kenya to change her laws and defy her family traditions by legalizing the killing of unborn children[63]; and pro-abortionists are promoting such proposals of anti-women and anti-child policies of abortion in order to decimate the Kenya population, and that to them, it was time that the Kenyan population rejected such birth control imperialism and defended the African tradition of love of the African family, and love of the child" He concluded, by saying that, "the Western nations is seen by the people to have developed their economic strength during periods of high population growth in the last century and that their attempts to decimate the Kenyan population by killing their children in the womb may suit their political and economic interests, but do nothing for the future of the Kenyan people."[64]

---

[62] Joni Seager, et al. 1997, Pp. 36.
[63] Thomas Lynn 1998, Pp. 121.
[64] I. Mutua, 'Why abortion is reprehensible', The African Law Review edited by Imanyara Gitobu. Issue 72, June 1998

In citing the Canada experience where abortion is legalized without any law indicating gestational limits; Anna Desilets, an executive director of the "Alliance for Life"- a pro-life group pointed out that, "easy access to abortion and contraception leads people to use it as birth control at tax payers expense. Her position was buttressed by a record high of 104,403 abortions performed in Canada in 1993, which was an indication of 2.3 percent increase over the previous year's, which amounted to 26.9 abortions per 100 live births. She attributed the increase to the, increasing number of private abortion clinics in the country as well as economic pressures."[65]

Some researchers also pointed out that, "many who can readily envision the concrete humanity of foetus, and hold its picture high and weep, barely see the woman who carries it and her plight ...and that many others, who can readily envision the woman and her body, who cry out for her right to control her destiny, barely envision the foetus within that woman and do not imagine as real the life it might have been allowed to lead."[66] It pointed out further, that while this moral issue rages on, from 50 million to 60 million unborn casualties will this year (i.e. in 1993) fall on the battlefield of rights.[67]

In the brewing controversy, the pro-life alliance upholds the right to life of all. They hinged their position on the Article 3, of the United Nations Declaration of Human Rights; which states 'that everyone has the right to life, liberty and security of persons'. Paradoxically, this same clause is being invoked by the pro-abortion advocates on the basis of legality, that women have a right not only to their bodies but as well as their security. The heat on this controversial issue of abortion, and contraception, erupted on February 1999, in Hague, Netherlands, when the head of the Holy See delegation, Monsignor Dewane Frank, delivered the Catholic's church paper that spoke of *'everyone's right to life.'* In supporting this view, he referred, to the misconception of the 1994 Cairo document on ' Population and Development ', "that in no case should abortion be promoted as a method of family planning". He denounced the present practice of emergency contraception and the use of the RU 486 pill for abortion camouflaged as contraception. He concluded that those means of contraception were contrary to the National legislative systems, which grant legal protection and safeguards to life from the moment of conception.[68]

Frances Kissling, the Catholics for a free choice president, reacted to Dewane's position in a rejoinder titled *'Religion: Getting Involved'*, that the Holy See tries to confuse the issue of abortion and contraception. She stated in her position further, that, "the Holy See sought to constrain women's freedom and confuse the issues, and that abortion and contraception are two different things. Pointing out

---

[65] Awake, 1996, Pp. 28.
[66] Tribe H. Lawrence, 1992, Pp. 93-96.
[67] Awake, 1993, Pp. 3.
[68] Daily Catholic News, 1999, Vol. 10, number 29.

that emergency contraception is a moral life saver for women as it prevents both pregnancy and abortion."[69]

While the issue of abortion and contraception attract debates, negotiations and controversy in other countries. The situation is contrary in China, Pakistan, Indian, Japan and Taiwan. In these countries, abortion and sometimes contraception, has become a comprehensive, package by their various governments for the control of population growth and socio-economic enhancement of the people as well as a policy to save the woman's, physical and mental health. With the population of China put at 1.2 billion people, and India's 1 billion people, more than thirty percent of the World's population is profoundly discriminated against by their government's draconian policies where abortion is regarded as fertility regulation and often as economic necessity. In Indian and Pakistan, there is forced abortion amongst young women. While in China, there is the forced one-child policy.[70] In 1978, there was an adoption of legislative measures by the government of China where the constitution of the country included the phrase that, "the State advocates and encourages family planning", and in 1980 new marriage laws contained clauses intended to stimulate fertility regulations; For example, encouraging late marriages, husband and wife being duty bound to practice family planning etc. This situation was re-emphasized in the China's 1982 constitution. It also included the crucial clause that "contraception, abortion and sterilization were to be provided free of charge; free choice of which contraceptive to use; induced abortion to be used as a back up in case of contraceptive failure. Great efforts were made to provide adequate services, and emphasis was placed on staffing health institutions with well trained personnel" (UN's case studies in Population Policy, 1989). This situation of forced and compulsory abortion in China accounts for over 14 million per year. While in Japan, women decorate tiny statues with bibs and toys in memory of their aborted children. The public has a high anxiety about birth control pills.

In this whole controversy, is the introduction of the feminist pro-abortion advocates position of discrimination in the idea and conception that abortion and contraception be used as family planning technique. In their argument, they highlighted the unfair perspective to this practice from the cultural angle. They conceived that the Oriental cultures and most other cultures in Africa like, Sudan and the Urhobo, Okpe, Bini, Itsekiri and the Yoruba speaking people in Nigeria has long valued sons over daughters. So, where both sex determination procedures and abortion are easily available, female foetuses are being aborted in large numbers, unbalancing male-female birth ratios.[71]

---

[69] The Earth Times 1999, Pp. 2.
[70] Jamali Bachar, 'Controversy brews over abortion issues' Pan African News Agency (PANA), Dakar, Senegal; February 11, 1999 B.P.4056
[71] Awake 1993, Pp. 7.

In effect, the roles that race, sex and ethnicity have played in abortion controversy should be examined in the light of the feminist movements position. Consequently, social policies should be directed at the public perception of both the feminist fight for legal abortions and the anti-abortion activist. In fact, the discussion of both pro-life and pro-choice activists should be focused on issues as parental consents and notification for parents of teenagers seeking abortion.[72]

Nomboniso, G. (1996), buttressed her position on the emotive and sensitive issue of abortion and contraception as a pro-abortionist defender from the inherent inadequacies of the socio-cultural system in South Africa. She stated that, "the issue is traversed with contradictions that arise out of our cultures, traditions, religions, and the complexities of a society based on patrilineal heritage". She noted that, "the need to protect the integrity of our bodies is part of a struggle for equality and changing unequal power relations, and that patrilineal constraints need to be understood within the wider context of patriarchal relations which subordinates women". She summed up her position by claiming that, "the legal frameworks and the ground-breaking gains made by the South African constitution will have little meaning if women are denied a choice that is intimate, private, personal and painful."[73]

In a polemical reaction to both the feminist and pro-abortion advocates of sex determination; Ferguson (1988) asserted that, "if the bill of pro-abortion advocates is a step towards women empowerment and only as an issue of women's liberation, then women have planted a seed of another cycle of oppression-one which neglects to hear that most silent voice of all, the voice of the unborn child". Furthermore, she said there was evidence that in Indian most abortions were of female foetuses. She asked, "Is this liberation of the woman? Is this what we are fighting for?"[74]

Arguing his position from both religious and socio-cultural angle, Father Marx Paul, a Professor of Sociology posited that, "abortion is the greatest killer of all times, it is World War III, and it is a war against those who have not been born."[75] He disagreed with the position that abortion could be a solution to the problem of over population and can establish the reproductive rights of the women. Rather, he outlined that abortion evokes a lot of problems such as the destruction of marriages, family life, prostitution; and that abortion is another desperate escapade by which immoral mothers and the young single girl tries to find a way out of her wrong deeds by covering up her unfaithfulness by killing and thus preventing the arrival of the undesired child within her." The ultimate question is; could this be true?

---

[72] R. T. Schaefer 1997, Pp. 343-346.
[73] Gasa-Suttner Nomboniso 1996, Pp. 18.
[74] A. Ferguson 1988, Pp. 74.
[75] Father Paul Marx 1998, Pp.3

While the controversy assumes a wider and more fierce dimension with a number of anti - abortion backlash reported in the United States between 1990-1995, there is an urgent need for a compromise situation that should be based on high sense of reasoning, rationality, and a down play of sentiments, emotions and socio-cultural value systems, particularly as it affects the adolescents or teenagers who are always in the process of adventurous seeking.

2.3. Abortion and Contraception: Comparison of Legal, Religious and Social Context in Nigeria

Abortion and contraception are out rightly outlawed by tradition, religion and statutory acts in Nigeria. In fact, the natural or unnatural death of an unborn baby is considered abortion. However, there is an acknowledgement of spontaneous abortions (miscarriages), which are considered natural occurrences. Consequently, if there is an outside assistance in whatever form to abort the baby, then it is believed that the murder of a God given life has taken place. It is the conviction of most cultures in Nigeria that 'abortion kills the life of the baby after it has begun'. It is in this light that abortion and contraception are seen as legal, religious, social and cultural offences by the perpetrators. Thus abortion is considered only necessary when there is a threat to the life of the pregnant woman (wanted or unwanted pregnancy).

The existing situation in Nigeria where access to contraception is restricted and abortion is regarded as illegal or 'highly restricted' to most women has resulted in the tremendous increase in unwanted pregnancies; particularly, with unsafe abortions, performed by untrained personnel in unhygienic conditions. Also, because most of the women living in rural areas have many pregnancies, the cumulative life risk of dying in pregnancy may reach an all time high.[76]

Otoide, V. (2000), summed it up in his paper on "Promoting Post-Abortion Care" as follows 'induced abortion is a complex and controversial subject that many people may not wish to acknowledge…the discomfort with the topics is due mainly to the fact that many people consider abortion to be morally wrong…this explains the position of the culture, tradition, religion and most importantly, the law on abortion in Nigeria and many developing countries, where induced abortion is illegal.'[77] In the absence of enabling laws, illegal and unsafe abortion, become the norm. Paradoxically, it is in these same countries that abortion takes its greatest toll on human lives and inflicts the greatest suffering.

Scholars posit that, many of the laws on reproduction applicable in most communities in Nigeria are customary and religious; and that women do not take

---

[76] Nigerian Vanguard Daily Newspaper 1998, Pp. 11.
[77] Valentine Otoide 2000, Pp. 1-4.

part in the enactment of these laws, chiefly as a result of cultural and religious constraints.[78]

In emphasizing the restriction in abortion and contraception adoption in Nigeria; The Post Express in 1999 reported on "Abortion: An Unmet Need", 'that abortion has been described as one of the factors indicating the ultimate unmet needs for family planning in Nigeria, because only a minority of women having abortions ever used effective contraception'. Presenting a report of data from a Contraceptive Prevalence Study (CPS) conducted by a group of researchers who are studying conditions of Nigerian women hospitalised for abortion complications, showed that most women would use contraceptives if they had access to them. The report however, noted that not all women who have had abortions would use contraception, rather many want to control their fertility in ways other than abortion, and only a minority of women agreed that their unmet need for contraception could be met, but they accepted that they could be helped to overcome barriers to contraceptive use.[79] This is a glaring awareness on display.

As a position against the twin practices of abortion and contraception, child marriages is common in most parts of Northern Nigeria. This is based on the erroneous belief that virginity can only be guaranteed between the ages of 8-10 years. It is also, hinged on the belief that it helps in forestalling promiscuity in young girls. It is further believed, that once a young girl has been packaged to her husband's house, she will not have time or space to be up to any mischief. In this regard, it is seen as a means of protecting family honour by preventing teenage pregnancy. In a study of the 'Nigerian Demographic and Health Survey in 1990, "it showed that among married female children sampled in Nigeria, the aggregate mean age at marriages is 16.7; and regional comparison indicate, that the lowest mean age at marriage are in the North-West which is put at 15.2 and 14.5. While in the Southern part the age for marriage is slightly higher. This situation has been attributed to the higher level of educational awareness in the Southern region". From the above position, it is a firm belief by the various cultures that early marriages tended to stem unwanted pregnancies, abortion and other forms of adolescents misdemeanours.

From both religious and socio-cultural perspectives, the practice of contraception and abortion in Nigeria is likened to slavery, which denies an individual his personhood.[80] The above position is further amplified by noting that conflict occurs between culture, which affirms, cherishes, and celebrates the gift of life; and another, which seeks to declare various groups of humans to be outside

---

[78] Theresa Akumadu 1997, Pp. 9.
[79] The Post Express News 1999, Pp. 1.
[80] Comments made by Chief Jon, a traditional herbalist and native doctor, on 'Abortion and female circumcision issues' during a personal interview at his residence which doubles as his traditional clinic, Sapele, October 15, 2000

boundaries of legal protection. Among these groups, they claim those yet unborn, the terminally ill, the handicapped and others considered non-useful.[81]

However, in trying to resolve the conflicting positions of the various interests on abortion and contraception, Johnson Diana in her paper titled *"Abortion: The French Solution",* stated that 'it is not surprising that different societies should have different ideas about sex; societies themselves change in their minds, even within a decade. More curious, maybe, is a difference in styles of democracy. Our society, seem to see the democratic process in confrontational terms, as a struggle of ideologies in which one finally defeats the other and imposes its view. France, however, see democracy as a process of workable compromises, even though no one is perfectly happy.'[82] In other words, whatever the differing views on the issue of abortion and contraception, all segment of the French society seem to agree on the collective goal-reducing the number of abortions.

In Nigeria, there is a lack of mechanism for consensus to share the goal of reducing the number of illegal abortions. There is equally a lack of a neutral entity for social decisions in general, a body (apart from the supreme court) whose matured reflections can be trusted to balance the completely intransigent factions and come up with workable policies. Whereas, we cannot achieve any social goal without controversy, in a case like this, involving health, it would mean acknowledging that the views of medical or educational experts are more germane than the sectarian concerns of clergymen or job security concerns of congressmen. For the moment it seem that polarized emotions rules over statistics, over medical expertise, over the experience of other societies and even over plain commonsense. In fact, religious leaders, media pundits and elected government officials have all squandered their authority and credibility on partisan politics and hypocritical moral posturing and we have never had the stable class of government functionaries that in Nigeria plays an important stabilizing role. These bureaucrats operate outside the strictly political arena, ignoring intemperate and inflexible factions on every side, plodding along with the public good in mind.[83]

2.4. Religion and Abortion

Religions are ideas and practices that symbolize a social group. It involves shared beliefs and practices that have a unifying effect in a social group. Thus, religion functions principally to create and maintain social solidarity.[84]

---

[81] The Post Express News 1999, Pp. 1.
[82] Diane Johnson, 'Abortion: The French solution' full text published in the editorial page of the Post Express newspaper online, February 2, 2000: www.postexpresswired.com, accessed on February 29, 2000.
[83] Ibid
[84] Onigu Otite and William Ogionwon 1981, Pp. 36.

In Nigeria, there exist three major forms of religious divisions; namely, the Christian, Islamic, and Traditional religions. They individually appeal to wide array of followers. Although, it is difficult to claim which of these religions have the most followers, it is incontrovertible that each is popular on its own form. More so, the Christian and Islamic religions are seen as imported religions embellished by the indigenous traditions and cultures of the people. Though, some skirmishes of other foreign minor religions like Hinduism, Buddhism, Guru Maharaji, Hare Krishna, etc exist, they are not too popular amongst the people, hence often regarded as inconsequential.

Whatever, the religion, there has existed throughout history, a diversity of opinion regarding the issue of abortion. "Today, there is no unanimity within various religions concerning a woman's right to chose abortion...women of every faith, even those with strict teachings against abortion have defied their religions in their reliance on abortion as a necessary means of ending unwanted pregnancies."[85] In the same vein, most people have used their religious denominations to anchor their points that 'committing abortion is against the precept and example of God.'

2.4.1. Christianity and Abortion

Early Christian condemned abortion but did not view the termination of a pregnancy to be an abortion before 'ensoulment'-the definition of when life began in the womb. Up to 400 AD, as the relatively few Christians were widely scattered geographically, the actual practice of abortion among Christians probably varied considerably and was influenced by regional customs and practices.[86]

Amongst the Urhobo, and Okpe speaking peoples of Nigeria, the most dominant Christian denominations are Catholic and Protestant churches. Though, there are other classified as Spiritual churches, Evangelical churches, Jehovah Witnesses etc. They all seem to be internally and deeply divided on the issue of abortion and contraception.

2.4.2. Roman Catholic Conception of Abortion

They consider contraception as intrinsically evil and they take the most rigid stance against abortion. They hold that abortion is never justified, and it is ground for excommunication under the church law. In fact, the church currents position against abortion stems from its moral and traditional practices, and has never been official doctrine or dogma.[87] However today, there is an internal opposition group to the position of the church. These are the group known as 'Catholics for free

---

[85] Jodi L. Jacobson 1990, Pp. 6-9.
[86] Deborah R. Mcfarlane 1993, Pp. 77-82.
[87] Jane Hurst 1983, Pp. 4-5.

Choice-Pro-choice Catholic groups'

2.4.3. Protestant Conception of Abortion

They are deeply divided on the issue of abortion. They repudiate in their statement what they call 'abortion on demand', but up-hold the sanctity of life, and set out means for ministering to women facing unwanted pregnancies. The Protestants however, agree on special circumstances on which abortion may take place.

2.4.4. Anglican Conception of Abortion

There are also some divisions on abortion policy in the Anglican churches of Nigeria. While one section of the congregation advocate on liberalization based on situation when the woman's life is endangered, the others out rightly condemn it.

Others like Baptist accept abortion when it endangers the life of the woman. While the Jehovah Witnesses, sees it as an out right sin to make life that one does not intend to care for, or at the same time to have an abortion.[88]

2.4.5. Islam and Abortion

Islamic doctrines affecting women and reproductive choice have more than one interpretation; and economic, political and social changes influences how Islam is translated into policies.[89] For instance the school of Islam, which permits the use of contraception is followed in many countries today; although, there are other schools which forbids its use. But the conservative school of Islam, which forbid abortion at any stage of pregnancy, is the one prevalent in majority of Arab countries.[90]

Specifically in Tunisia (since 1965) and Turkey (since 1983), abortion is considered legal under another interpretation of Islam. While in Jordan and Egypt, as in the rest of the Arab countries, abortion is illegal, with a few medical exceptions.[91] However, in Nigeria, Islamic scholars of the two main sects (many of whom are, Sunni and Shites) agree that abortion at or after the 'ensoulment stage' is prohibited, except to save the life of the woman.

2.4.6. Tradition and Abortion

Traditionally, abortion amongst the Urhobo, Okpe, Isoko, Hausa, Yoruba and Bini ethnic groups in Nigeria is considered killing of life. Contradictorily, it is the same tradition that creates circumstances and situations that encourages back alley abortions, because of its social demand. Although, children from unwanted pregnancies are often, adopted by other members of the extended family or

---

[88] Awake 1993, Pp. 8.
[89] Carla Makhlouf Obermeyer 1994, Pp. 25-51.
[90] El-Sadawi Nawal 1990, "Views from the Arab World: Woman must own her body" IPPF, Vol. 17, no. 4.
[91] Nahid Toubia 1994, Pp. 21.

community, such children often suffer negative social stigma. More so, many traditions and culture like the Urhobo, Okpe and Igbo speaking people tend to force young women to seek abortion, as there are strong social sanctions against unmarried women with children, and an unmarried pregnant woman without a suitor could be ostracized, disowned by her relatives or looked upon as a dreg in the society.[92]

2.5. Adolescents and Abortion

The issue of reproductive health and sexual behaviour has its greatest impact and victims on adolescents. The Population Reference Bureau (PRB) research on the 'World's Youths in 1996', revealed that unintended pregnancies among teens account for at least 2 million unsafe abortions occurring among women ages 15-19. It also mentioned that the proportion of abortion occurring in many countries appears to be rising; and that adolescents are less likely than other women to use contraception, resulting in higher rate of unintended pregnancies. Furthermore, it pointed out that in much of the developing world, access to legal abortion is severely restricted, leading millions of women to resort to unsafe procedures; and that young women are more likely to hide their pregnancies and seek clandestine abortion services later in their pregnancies, further increasing the associated health risk.[93] In fact, women and adolescent females resort to illegal and unsafe abortion for a number of reasons. These include fear of not meeting societal and familial expectations, strict anti-abortion laws, lack of financial and health resources, a desire not to have a baby, lack of knowledge of sexuality and reproductive health, and misinformation from peers and adults alike.[94]

The World Health Organization (WHO) estimates that, 'between 40-60 million abortions are performed annually worldwide out of which an estimated 20 million are unsafe. It stated further, that at least eighty thousand women die each year as a result and many more experience life long physical and mental health problems as a result of unsafe abortion. It further revealed that most of the unsafe abortions are performed outside the health care system, by unskilled providers and under unsanitary conditions. It identified sex among unmarried young people as a major factor in the significant number of these abortions. The report concluded that, with increased modernity and exposure of young people, pre-marital sex has become more common among young people, where substantial numbers of them have their first sexual experience outside marriage

In Nigeria, the trend is a typical reflection of the report of the PRB. In SIECUS International program 1996, it revealed that, Nigerian adolescents continue to account for 80 percent of abortions treated in Nigerian hospitals annually. One

---

[92] Babatunde Suleiman 1993, Pp. 1
[93] J. Noble, J. Cover, and M. Yanagishita, "The World's Youth 1996"-Popualtion Reference Bureau, 1996, Pp. 1-2.
[94] Valentine Otoide 2000, Pp.4

out of every four sexually active teenage girl in Nigeria has procured at least one abortion and more than half of these procedures; were carried out by non-professional providers. This growing trend of unsafe abortion among adolescents has been described as a ' school girls problem' in Nigeria today.[95]

The 1996 Population Reference Bureau studies suggested that meeting the contraceptive needs of sexually experienced youth is one of the most effective ways of lowering the incidence of abortion; as well as providing non-punitive and high quality post-abortion care which includes contraceptive information and counselling for girls and their partners. It stated that if some of these conditions could be provided, it would help to improve adolescent health as well as lower the incidence of repeat abortion. Complementing the suggestion of the PRB; A research study was of the opinion that, pending the achievement of the cardinal goal (liberalized abortion), there is need to implement a broad strategy that seeks to reduce the incidence of unprotected sexual exposure and unwanted pregnancies amongst adolescents...that there is need to promote sex education, especially of adolescents, promote responsible sexual behaviour and encourage contraceptive use for the prevention of unwanted pregnancies.[96] In addition, he recommended that health providers should in like manner be educated on the provision of abortion and post-abortion contraception to break the circle of repeat abortions common amongst adolescents in the country (Nigeria).

---

[95] O. Odujirin 1996, Pp. 361-362.
[96] Valentine Otoide 2000, Pp. 4.

3.0. Chapter three
3.1. Female Circumcision, Cultural Mutilation and Identity

Cross cultural body modification, other wise known as mutilation, has always been a constant cultural features of most existing cultures in the world. Cultural mutilation has been done for the purpose of identity. Thevoz Michel in his book, "*The Painted Body*" tried to explain the origin of cultural mutilation as a form of cultural identity.[97] He expanded upon Louis Bolk's concept that "humans are biologically incomplete creatures as compared with other mammals, and that the absence of fur, facial reduction, vertical brow and large cranial volume are signs of "persistent foetalisation" that includes a loss of instincts as a consequence of this adaptation. Thus the human being according to him is born disinherited from the animal kingdom and dependent on the care of parents for years. He is also, born naked-exposed to danger and the surveillance of others. 'The self-retouching impulse, which is another word for his description of mutilation, was originated by man out of the awareness of this biological incompleteness to further distinguish humans from other animal; and the need to invent culture in order, to deny natural determinism'. Consequently, meaningful body modification is viewed as a way through which the individual establishes his identity and social status in the practising society. This is believed to help ensure social order.

Thevoz noted that the precedence for early tool making was symbolic for the purpose of magic and the need to create a body culture. In this context, mutilation was not seen as cruelty or inhuman, since it was done on cultural basis even with its noticeable physical and health complications.

Advocates of cultural mutilation argue that the term 'mutilation' entails negative connotation of an action based on intents. In other words, mutilation becomes it when people inject emotions into cultural actions or facts. To such advocates, cultural mutilation served the purpose of maintaining social order. In fact, scarification was probably the commonest form of cultural mutilation in many African cultures. It is found among many groups in West, Central, and East Africa - for example, Nuba, Nri, Dinka, Tiv, Yoruba, Urhobo, Hausa.[98] Typically, cuts are made for beautification and ritual purposes. Linear scars, and round cuts are produced by deep cuts with sharp instruments like small razor blade and knives to produce permanent scar. Keloids formation is often the desired results. The ritual explanation is that these scars enforce group affiliations and promote tribal integration. The marks vary from tribe to tribe. Even the American Indians were noted for the mutilation of their heads, while in the time past, the Japanese aristocracy mutilated women's leg from when they were young.

---

[97] Michel Thevoz 1984, Pp. 45-46.
[98] R. C. Desrosiers 1986, Pp. 319.

Cultural apologist like Nowa Omoigui liken female circumcision to western form of body mutilations like tattooing, Piercing and silicon implantation which she refer to as a form of bodily mutilation to achieve or attain beauty of the woman. She wondered why there is a focus on female circumcision when there are so many other dangerous forms of western cultural mutilations that require attention. She questioned why female circumcision is special? This is evident in her argument in a work titled 'Protest Against Bill HB22 Outlawing 'FGM' in Nigeria' she argued further "...who advised the World Health Organization to coin the phrase 'mutilation'? Whoever did, was cynically manipulating language. We 'mutilate' the umbilical cord by cutting it off at birth and arbitrarily deciding how long the navel should be. We "mutilate" our bodies with earrings, tongue rings, tattoos, nose jobs etc. We 'keep' biologically excretory products like nails and hair, and use them for beautification and do so differently, I might add, depending on the cultural environment. Some western women (in the US) begin to shave their leg hair at age 10. They also shave their armpits. Has anyone else in the world attacked them for mutilating what God put there for a reason? We use traditional scarification marks for medicinal and symbolic purposes... some of which result in disfiguring keloids. Why is that not 'mutilation' of the skin? Why not ban it? Why then female circumcision?"[99]

Antagonists of female circumcision hold that most of all the forms of bodily mutilations particularly, scarification are gradually been done away with because of the accompanying health hazard and modernization. More so, they argue that whether it is mutilation for beauty or for cultural purpose, the idea is that female circumcision is inimical to health; and the idea itself is propelled by a 'schizo-paranoid impulse'[100], such as anarchy, cannibalism, incest, destruction and murder; and that is the underlying manifest explanations for justifying the call for its discontinuity.[101]

3.2. Female Circumcision as Cultural Violence

Female circumcision otherwise known as female genital mutilation (FGM) is regarded as "good tradition" in areas where it is still effectively practiced throughout the world. However, recent studies has detailed and documented serious and un-measurable reproductive and sexual health complications associated with this practice that is still common in most parts of Africa, the Middle - East, and Asia. Today, the complications associated, with this practice has made it a global conscious public health concern that requires legislation to curb its continuous practice. With the number of global victims put at about 130 million women today, it is no doubt one of the greatest sexual health horrors.

---

[99] Nowa Omoigui, 2001, Pp.8.
[100] The sudden impulse by a person with mental disorder to act or reason irrationally or abnormally
[101] Michel Thevoz 1984, Pp. 46.

Even, the highest maternal and infant mortality rates have been identified in female genitally mutilated practicing regions of the world.[102]

The major thrust of this research on female circumcision is the concern of this unfortunate practice among many ethnic groups in Nigeria, with an estimated population of the of over 55 million women scattered over about 350 existing ethnic groups, and the overall national prevalence rate of the practice put at about fifty percent, and thus accounts for the highest absolute number of genitally mutilated women throughout the world, yet there is no legislation in place to curb the practice.[103]

In the practicing regions (areas) in Nigeria, female circumcision is somewhat, autocratic and downright condescending amongst the people. The age long tradition is not only medieval in its approach but also popular among the practitioners. This has made the issue to be more than serious when weighed along the inherent dangers associated with its perpetuation. Today the issue that has become a 'socio - medical phenomenon.'[104] What is at stake is no longer an issue for women's right alone but that of public and global decency, and the health of all females in practising communities.

3.3. The Politics of Culture and Female Circumcision

The idea that female circumcision is an age long tradition and cultural practice of the people has been used as its 'sustainability theory' by its advocates. Some other advocates have used Christianity and Islam to argue that the practice be continued even when they are no clear basis to support such in the doctrines. The female victims of this cultural violence are either under or over aged. All of this is strictly, dependent on the upheld variability that exists amongst ethnic groups in relation to the practice. Reasons for the continuation of female circumcision ranges from religious requirements, rites of passage to womanhood, virginal cleanliness, prevention of promiscuity amongst girls, better marriage prospects, enhancement of male sexuality, prevention of excessive clitoral growth, to facilitation of the childbirth by widening of the birth canal.[105] In Okpe, Urhobo, Bini, Ika and Isoko communities among many others in Nigeria where female circumcision are still held as sacred, the practice is regarded as a good tradition.[106]

Also, the patriarchal nature of the Urhobo, okpe and Isoko ethnic groups in Nigerian imposes a stigma on the girl child by relegating her to a subordinate position. For instance, violence against girls was all about male power dominance and control in these societies. It is, also, about the control of language values that socializes the boys to think and hold the belief that women are

---

[102] Fran P. Hosken 1993, Pp. 37.

[103] Mairo U. Mandara 1995, Pp. 29-36.

[104] Female circumcision is now an issue that has attracted both social and medical concern of advocates for its abolition in practising communities.

[105] M. D. Calverton 1989/1990, Pp. 118.

[106] Fran P. Hosken 1993, Pp. 3.

owned, by them as properties. Thus they grow into men to put all these conceptions and values into practice. This explains particularly, the reason why women are more vulnerable, 'they could be seen but not to be heard.' This vulnerability of women to socio-cultural, legal and religious issues limits them from taking decisions or being part of decisions on matters that concern them. Thus, it bestows on men the responsibilities and /or such concerns to carry on the fight for women's rights. This socio-cultural barrier makes it difficult for women to express their disgust openly on unhealthy reproductive health practices like female circumcision. Unfortunately, some women who could have been in a better position to resist paternalistic traditional framework compromise their positions under the guise of moral arguments, thereby forgetting that they are assisting in promoting male sexuality in their ignorant quest to protect cultural values and morality in which they have little or no rights. Feminist writer, Germaine Greer in her recent book "The Whole Woman" defended stoutly the perpetuation of female circumcision in practicing countries. She argued, that attempts to outlaw the practice of FGM amounted to an attack on 'cultural identity' of practicing countries. In her words,

> "Looked at in its full context the criminalization of FGM can be seen to be what African nationalists since Jomo Kenyatta have been calling it, an attack on cultural identity. Any suggestion that male genital mutilation should be outlawed would be understood to be a frontal attack on the cultural identity of Jews and Muslims. Notwithstanding, the opinion that male circumcision might be bad for babies, bad for sex and bad for men is steadily gaining ground. In Denmark only 2 percent of non-Jewish and non-Muslim men are circumcised on strictly non-medical grounds; in Britain the proportion rises to between 6 percent and 7 percent, but in the U.S. between 60 percent and 70 percent of male babies will have their foreskins surgically removed. No UN agency has uttered a protocol condemning the widespread practice of male genital mutilation, which will not be challenged until doctors start to be sued in large numbers by men they mutilated as infants. Silence on the question of male circumcision is evidence of the political power both of the communities where a circumcised penis is considered an essential identifying mark and of the practitioners who continue to do it for no good reason. Silence about male mutilation in our own countries combines nicely with noisiness on female mutilation in other countries to reinforce our notions of cultural superiority."[107]

However, her sense of sanctity of culture has been, attacked by various groups and organizations as simplistic and offensive in the light of her failure not to take account of the purposes of female genital mutilation, nor the lack of choice of young people in deciding on issues that affects them directly; for instance, parental influence on spouse selection common among the Urhobo and Okpe speaking ethnic groups of Nigeria and many ethnic groups in Kenya. Nowa Omoigui, argued in support of Greer that if choice of the girl were necessary then she should be made to grow up and take decisions on other very crucial issues that concerns them. She summed it up in this format, "A common argument among proponents of HB22 and similar legislation is that children

---

[107] Germaine Greer 1999, Pp. 102.

(rather than their parents) be allowed to make the decision whether to get circumcised when they get to age 18. In my view, this suggestion amounts to a pervasive interference in the right of families to rear their children in their own cultural and religious likeness. The 'let children grow up and decide' argument can equally apply to all other aspects of life. Let them grow up and decide whether and what schools to attend; what religion to practice; whether to cut their hair, pierce their ears, shave their armpits, shave their legs; what foods to eat; what language to speak, etc. They might even have the right to divorce their parents - as occurred in Florida recently. But the more one travels along this curious line of reasoning the farther away from our essence as Africans one gets."

However, Lightfoot-Klein in her argument against Greer and Omoigui position in her book: 'Prisoner of Ritual: An Odyssey into Female Genital Circumcision in Africa.' hold that;

> "The reasons given for female circumcision in Africa and for routine male circumcision in the U.S. are essentially the same. Both falsely tout the positive health benefits of the procedures. Both promise cleanliness and the absence of "bad" genital odours, as well as greater attractiveness and acceptability of the sex organs. The affected individuals in both cultures have come to view these procedures as something that was done for them and not to them…Childhood genital mutilations are anachronistic rituals inflicted on the helpless bodies of non-consenting children of both sexes."[108]

This position of Greer is seen in the context, as sounding a global cautionary notes that, it is important for western organizations to ensure that campaigns against female genital mutilation is not seen as trying to impose western cultural value judgement upon the culture of practicing ethnic groups but to support the numerous grassroots and community organizations engaged in campaigns to eradicate the practice, least they are accused of being racists or disrespectful (Mohammad, R. 1999: 5)

Some advocates noted that 'when the perceived benefits or cultural relevance of female genital mutilation are weighed against the health complications, the scale of medical opinion clearly support its abolition.[109] This is because though custom in some of its intricate forms has drastic consequences for women's health, sexuality and fertility, it also has serious medical complications on the health of the woman.' Though, some health practitioners have used medical technology to improve some aspects of those customs, which reduces trauma during the procedure and infection afterwards, they claimed (medical experts) that this does not address female circumcision long term consequences for childbearing and sexuality and that culture and tradition should not be used as an excuse for inaction in securing women's rights.[110] He held further that, "The unnecessary

---

[108] Hanny Lightfoot-Klein 1997, Pp. 193.
[109] Valentine Otoide 2000, Pp. 3-4.
[110] Nahid Toubia 1994, Pp. 127-135.

removal of a functioning body organ in the name of tradition, custom or any other non-disease related cause should never be acceptable to the health profession. All childhood circumcisions are violations of human rights and a breach of the fundamental code of medical ethics. It is the moral duty of educated professionals to protect the health and rights of those with little or no social power to protect themselves."

In that respect, culture is viewed as dynamic and subject to changes; and people are urged to have a choice in formulating the constituents of their cultural and religious fallacies and dichotomies. In other words, the ultimate verdict of a perceived cultural wrong cannot even be solely passed by the court of law, but in the court of public opinion, that encompasses, both the victims, communities, men, governments, and the entire society.

3.4. The Legal Violation of Female Circumcision in Nigeria

The World Health Organization (WHO) and the United Nations Children Fund (UNICEF), acknowledges that, the girl child as well as the global woman have rights of their own. Indeed, they hold that female genital mutilation is an abuse of the rights of the girl child and have enjoined all countries to discontinue the practice. The legal and human rights frameworks on their part, and in their effort to eradicate the practice of FGM has as its, implicit constitutional consideration, the idea and notion that the rights of the girl child is incontrovertible. Undoubtedly, female genital mutilation is an encroachment on the physical and 'psycho-sexual' integrity of women and thus, constitutes a form of violence against them.

In drawing attention to some of the globally recognized provisions in the United Nations declarations on the rights of the girl child: article 5 of the United Nations Declaration of Human Rights submit that "...no one shall be subjected to torture or cruel inhuman or degrading treatment". Also, the United Nations Declaration on the Elimination of Violence against Women (General Assembly resolution 48/104, 1993) and the Platform for Action of the Forth World Conference on Women (Beijing 1995) stated that, " violence against women both violates, impairs and nullifies the enjoyment of their human rights and fundamental freedom". At the Continental level, article 21 of the African Charter on the Rights and Welfare of the Child, emphasizes, "...that appropriate measures be taken in order to eradicate traditional practices and customs which are prejudicial to the child". Despite the ratifications of these provisions by most member countries of the U.N. and O.A.U., no effective action has been taken to address these anomalies in Nigeria. Even the Commonwealth Jurisdiction enacted laws specifying female circumcision as maiming or wounding. With all these in place, most member countries including Nigeria have also, failed to put effective structures in place to legislate against female genital mutilation. Rather, the Nigerian government and her agents have continued to frustrate the series of efforts to legislate against the practice by inventing all forms of technicalities which are hinged on the usual traditional, cultural, religious and moral reasons.

38

To amplify this point, only recently, the mass media reported that the lower house of the National Assembly in Nigeria threw out a bill-captioned 'HB22 outlawing FGM in Nigeria' that was initiated to legislate against the practice of female circumcision on technical grounds. Although, there have been piecemeal legislations against the practice in some states of the Nigeria federation like Edo, Delta and Ogun.[111] It is considered, by many that only more national concern and consensus could prove effective in the campaign against female circumcision. Unfortunately, most women who stand in advantage position to fight against the continuous practice are the greatest conspirators in the name of religion, tradition, culture, morality and survival.[112]

The raging controversies between those who are advocates for and against the practice of female circumcision raises fundamental questions, such as, whether the right to preserve cultural and religious practices should take precedence over the health complications and the international enormity of the human rights of the girl child? Or whether culture should not be allowed to serve the purpose that it is meant in practising ethnic groups?

3.5. Female Circumcision as Symbolic Ritual

Rituals are repeated pattern of behaviours performed at appropriate times, and which may involve the use of symbols. Durkheim in his work on "The Elementary Forms of the Religious Life, 1912) categorised rituals firmly as sacred rather than profane. He reduced ritual to social structure and argued that rituals create social solidarity. For him the unit of significance in ritual is action, since action causes beliefs, not vice versa.

Amongst the Urhobo and Okpe speaking ethnic groups in Nigeria, female circumcision is conceived as a form of spiritual cleansing of the female. The circumcised female is made to undergo a period of seclusion during which she recovers and provided with the tribal knowledge on sexuality, procreation and how to relate with their future husband. These rites also, mark initiation into adulthood, marriage, and death, as well as entrance into various special groups (e.g. holding of Chieftaincy title, which is considered a political traditional title). Among the Ijaw speaking people of the Niger Delta and the Igbo speaking people of eastern Nigeria the transition from girl to womanhood is mark by female circumcision.[113]

Ritually, the shedding of blood during female circumcision has a spiritual implication for the Urhobo and Okpe speaking ethnic groups. It is believed that it made it right for the woman to conceive and procreate. Uncircumcised girls were

---

[111] Chinwe Okoronkwo 'Groups advocates bill against genital mutilation' in the Guardian online: www.ngrguardiannews.com, Sunday, July 1, 2001; and Austin Ogwuda 'Delta moves against female circumcision' in the Vanguard online: www.vanguardngr.com.

[112] Gbemi Egunjobi, 'What do you know about women' in the Guardian online: www.ngrguardiannews.com, Sunday, June 10, 2000.

[113] Onigu Otite and William Ogionwon 1981, Pp. 263.

considered ritually unclean and cannot participate in some cultural events and activities. For example she cannot cook for her husband or man to eat or belonged to a prominent woman social group called the 'Ewe ya.'[114] She is stigmatised and treated as an outcast. Even the acceptance of a bride-wealth of an uncircumcised girl or woman was considered a curse. Female circumcision among the Urhobo and Okpe people is accompanied with elaborate rituals, and ceremonies. For instance, lavish cooking after successful mutilation along with gift giving to the girl (victim) and members of her family. Specifically, among the Urhobo people, the woman or girl's body was coloured with a red like traditional cream, while family members wore dotted native chalks on their forehead as a mark of identification of a new initiate by way of circumcision in the family. It is the belief of the people that a person is not just born into society, but has to be recreated through, the rites of passage, as a social individual, and accepted into society, and for them this process for Urhobo, Okpe, Isoko and Bini speaking ethnic groups in Nigerian is through female circumcision.

3.6. Religion and Female Circumcision

There are conflicting views regarding the place of female circumcision in religious interpretation. A large number of people from the southern and northern parts of Nigeria practice female circumcision as tradition required and supported by Christian and Islamic religions even when there are no clear basis in any of these religious precepts for the practice of female circumcision in the Bible and Koran. However, female circumcision among practicing ethnic groups in the two regions has been known to predate both religions. A common argument by both religions for the sustenance of the practice has been that a 'non-excised or circumcised woman is impure in a religious sense.'

3.7. Christianity and Female Circumcision

The imputation of the Christian religion in culture as interpretation of female circumcision among the Urhobo and Okpe speaking peoples of Sapele and Ethiope-east local government areas respectively is embellished by the non-condemnation of the practice by the predominant orthodox Christian denominations- the Catholic and Anglican churches in these areas. They adopt non-condemnation of the practice as a strategy to retain their adherents and believers, since they were not prepared to lose both their believers and the accompanying economic benefits (tithes) that accrues the churches as it were when they took an earlier stance against the practice because of the health complications. Thus the orthodox churches, in these areas have adapted over time through liberal attitudes and ideas in their teachings to the tradition of the people and accommodated the practice of female circumcision.

---

[114] 'Ewe Ya' is an association of women commonly found in Okpe and Urhobo speaking areas. They play prominent role in the social and political structure of the community. Women members must be excised to belong.

However, with the emergence of fundamental Christian sects of new generation churches in these areas, liberal attitudes and religious diplomacy in teaching towards the custom of female circumcision and other reproductive health issues was transformed to radical doctrines which came out with 'unclear biblical' support for female circumcision, and condemned the use of contraceptives and abortion. Some of the confusion, which may have arisen with regard to these fundamental Christian religious sects and their interpretations of the Bible is probably due to generalization from male circumcision to female.[115]

Although, excision and infibulation is practiced by many Moslems in the Northern part of Nigeria through the imposition of Islamic fundamentalist doctrine and the Sharia legal system in Zamfara, Kaduna, Kano, Kebbi, Sokoto, Bornu, Yobe, Jigawa states. The excision form is practiced mainly by, Catholics, Protestants, and Anglican Christians in the Southern part of Nigeria especially among the Igbos of the South-east, and the Urhobo, Okpe, and the Isoko of the Delta area.

In both religions, religious scholars, academics and researchers have found no strong and clear basis in Christian and Islamic doctrines on the practice of female circumcision.

3.8. Female Circumcision and the contraction of HIV/AIDS

There are controversies in research and scholarly circles on the relationship between female circumcision and the contraction of the dreaded Human Immunodeficiency Virus (HIV) and the Acquired Immune Deficiency Syndrome (AIDS). Some scholars argue, that there is lack of correspondence of the distribution of AIDS and female circumcision. This group hold that 'infibulations occur mainly in the Arabian Peninsula, isolated areas of West Africa, the Horn of Africa, the Sudan and Northern Kenya areas, but yet it is not corroborated with the AIDS transmission.'[116] These individuals also hold the views that if female circumcision is an important determinant of AIDS transmission, it is difficult to understand why parts of Central Africa, South Africa, where the levels of AIDS are highest and where AIDS was first described do not practice female circumcision.[117]

Others presuppose that such harmful cultural practices like female circumcision could predispose the individual to the HIV/AIDS infection because of the mode of operation that is often very traditional and unhygienic. Their argument is further based on the medical perspective which state that since female circumcision leads on a regular basis to wounds and infections in the genitals, every circumcised woman is much more likely to get infected with the HIV-virus during the first intercourse with an infected man.

---

[115] Efua Dorkenoo 1995, Pp. 36-39.
[116] Pierrette Herzberger-Fofana, paper delivered and discussions on ‚Gewalt und Sexualität in der afrikanischen Frauenliteratur: Die Auseinandersetzung um Genitalverstümmelung' on May 15, 2001, at Institüt für Soziologie, FU-Berlin.
[117] Daniel B. Hrdy 1987, Pp. 1109.

41

Daniel, B. H. (1987) in his work on 'Cultural Practices Contributing to the Transmission of HIV in Africa' states that "differences between the epidemiology of AIDS cases in Africa and that in the Western societies have prompted speculations regarding risks factors that may be unique to Africa. Because of the age and sex distribution of AIDS in Africa, emphasis has been placed on the sexual transmission of HIV.[118] Factors thought to influence this sexual transmission include, promiscuity, with a high prevalence of sexually transmitted disease; sexual practices that have been associated with increased transmission of AIDS virus (homosexuality and anal intercourse); and cultural practices that are possibly connected with increased virus transmission (female circumcision and infibulations). Other non-sexual cultural practices that do not fit the age distribution pattern of AIDS but may expose individuals to HIV include; practices resulting in exposure to blood (medicinal blood letting, rituals establishing "blood brotherhood"); practices involving the use of shared instruments (injection of medicines, ritual scarification, group circumcision, genital tattooing, and shaving of body hair); and contact with non-human primates.

Other researchers postulates that female circumcision, increase the likelihood of AIDS transmission via increased exposure to blood in the vaginal canal.[119] The presumed explanation is that the small introituses, the presence of scar tissue (which may cause tissue friability), and the abnormal anatomy of a mutilated vaginal would predispose to numerous small (or large) tears in the mucosa during intercourse. These tears would tend to make the squamous vaginal epithelium similar in permeability to the columnar mucosa of the rectum, which increase absorption of secretions (and virus). A less likely explanation involves sexual intercourse shortly at or after the time of female circumcision, when open wounds are present. Corroborating the above position, Brady (1999) reports, that in one of the conferences on possible HIV transmission, a research study performed in Nairobi indicated that female circumcision predisposes women to HIV infection in many ways (for example, increase need for blood transfusion due to haemorrhage either when the procedure is performed, at childbirth, or a result of vaginal tearing during de-infibulations and intercourse, and the use of the same instruments for other initiates).[120] Because female circumcision raises the social status of the parents, the dowry demands can be high and therefore, the young girl can be married off to older men who are already infected.[121]

Consequently, questions relating to female circumcision and the HIV/AIDS require further researches for a concrete scientific explanation. There is the need to know the distribution of population groups (that is, tribes) that have high rates

---

[118] Ibid, Pp.1109
[119] R. A. Mannes 1985, Pp.623-626
[120] Margaret Brady 1999, Pp. 709-710.
[121] C. Oyugi 1998, Pp. 12.

of sero- positivity correlate with the distribution of groups that practice female circumcision.

3.9. Factors that aid Female Circumcision Practice in Nigeria

A number of factors help in fostering the continuous practice of FGM in Nigeria. Prominent amongst such factors are:

• Gender-based discrimination. That is an important determinant of poor reproductive health of women. Thus women suffer the major burden of sexual and reproductive ill health because they encounter discrimination in access to basic needs, health services and the exercise of human rights. Nature is not left out in the gender bias against women. This is so because nature ensures through what is a blind adherence to tradition, the basic explanation for the perpetuation of female circumcision. This course is embellished by, the strong patriarchal traditional institutional framework that is deeply rooted in many ethnic speaking groups 'socio-cultural structure' in Nigeria. Unfortunately, this course is defended by some women under the guise of morality; thereby forgetting that they assist in promoting male sexuality in their ignorant quest to protect cultural values and morality in which they have little or no rights.

• Negligence on the part of government to enact effective legislation in line with established UN and Continental Human Rights Conventions to protect women and children from cruelty and violence and ensure them bodily integrity and access to health care, education and self-realization.

• The neglect of the rural areas which is home to about three-quarter of the women population in Nigeria, and where FGM is deeply rooted and predominantly practiced in the enlightenment process against the traditional surgical practice of FGM.

• The non-inclusion of traditional opinion, and religious leaders in the process of mobilization and the enlightenment of the people against FGM, in order to expunge the superstitious beliefs that wraps, FGM in their world-view.

• The lack of awareness on the part of perpetrators who adopt, use and abuse religious injunctions to support or justify the practice of FGM.

3.10 What is to be Done?

In order to stem the tide of the practice of FGM and forestall the traditional and cultural injustices and criminality perpetuated against the girl child in Nigeria, there remains an imperative need for a systematic approach to address every aspect of the practice in order to provide a substantive and concerted framework for target intervention. Although, it is the researchers view and conviction that the major approach for tackling the practice FGM remains effective enlightenment, education and legislation; Within this context, the primary aim is to target and examine the following,

• who should be educated?
• who should do the educating?
• how and when should the education be imparted?

- what factors should exert a bearing on formulation of policies and legislation on the practice of FGM?
- how can these be sensitively and effectively, influenced to evolve a positive attitude and a constructive and sustained initiative on the part of policy makers?

These factors can help in the identification of the specific areas and mechanisms for target intervention on the part of policy formulators, as well as impact positively, on the behaviour and attitude of societal members towards the practice of FGM. It would also, create an avenue for promoting communication and sensitising women in particular, and society in general, on issues of women sexual disempowerment and the adverse consequences of this on the sexual reproductive health and well-being of women.

4.0. Chapter four
4.1. HIV and AIDS Infection in Nigeria
Nigeria has the fourth worst infection level of HIV/AIDS in Sub-Saharan Africa, with an estimated 3 million people infected, it is claimed that about 1.7 million people have died since the country's first AIDS case was diagnosed in 1986. The spread of the virus in Nigeria is accelerating with prevalence among adults in 1999 estimated at triple the rate measured in 1991 and general AIDS awareness remains low.[122] Specifically, HIV/AIDS prevalence in the country has increased from 5.4 percent to 5.8 percent in recent period. This increase showed that some of the interventions currently in place were not having the desired effect.

The HIV/AIDS scourge is not just a health concern but also has socio-economic implications for the country. For instance, the disease has erased a quarter century of increased life expectancy, bringing it back to about 47 years. It is also estimated to be costing the country 0.5 percent of per capital growth a year. In other words, the epidemic since it began has killed million of adults, decimated the work force, fractured and impoverished families, orphaned million of children, shredded the fabric of communities and worst still now invading the adolescents and youth population who are more vulnerable at this stage of human development. Globally, half of all new HIV/AIDS infections have been reported to occur in the 15-24 age groups, with an additional 6,000 young adults becoming infected every day.[123]

4.2. Adolescents, STD's and, HIV \ AIDS   Infections

SIECUS International program (1997: 16) in one of her reports stated that, "even though the level of sexual activity among young people is very high, the knowledge about safe sexual practice among them is poor". The World Health Organization (WHO), reports that the highest rates of STD's occur among 20-24 years old, followed by teens ages 15-19. It went further to reveal that HIV is spreading rapidly among young women ages 15-24. In many countries, women now account for 40 percent of all new HIV infections. On the average, women are becoming infected with HIV at ages 5-10 years younger than men.[124]

Researches on African countries have shown that cultural factors also help in putting adolescents at risk of contracting an STD, because they tend to engage in short-term sexual relationships and do not protect themselves from infections through contraceptives usage. Similarly, cultural factors make women vulnerable to STD's. For example, in some parts of Northern Nigeria and other African

---

[122] Raymond Toye, "World Bank Supports AIDS programmes in Nigeria, Burkina Faso." Washington, July 6, 2001; News Release No: 2002/005/Afr. And World Bank Report 2002, "Reversing the spread of HIV/AIDS: The youths hold the key" in www.worldbank.org/AIDS accessed on 8.07.2002

[123] The New York Times, "AIDS may kill up to 70 million, say UN." July 3, 2002 Pp. A19

[124] UNAIDS 1999, Pp. 5-8.

countries like, Kenya, Malawi, Uganda, Burundi etc. where younger women are paired with older men, they are more likely to become infected because older men have had more partners and younger women are less able to negotiate the use of contraception or other forms of contraceptives usage. In upholding the above assertion, a European study estimated that women were about twice as likely to get HIV from, an infected partner. In addition, young women exposed to HIV prior to genital maturation face a greater risk of infection due to physical immaturity of their reproductive system, and that since women are more likely than men to have an untreated STD because many STD's (like gonorrhoea, chlamydia) do not cause symptoms in women, the presence of either type of STD often increase the risk of HIV transmission as much as three to five fold as in the case in South Africa.

4.3. Adolescent and other Culturally Harmful Reproductive and Sexual Health Behaviours in Africa

In Africa, there are other very serious and harmful reproductive and sexual behaviours that affect and undermine the health of adolescent females much more than abortions, STD's, HIV and AIDS contraction.

Lukumbo, (1998) commenting on harmful practices in reproductive health disclosed that some communities in Tanzania actually elongate the clitoris instead of chopping it off as practiced in most countries where female genital mutilation (FGM) or circumcision is performed. According to him, young girls are introduced to Female Genital Elongation (FGE) on attainment of puberty by continuously being encouraged to pull the clitoris until it is long enough to cover the vagina.[125] He explained that this is done not only to help the man enjoy sexual intercourse but also to prevent rape. He pointed out further, that the act of pulling the organ is usually painful-which is why, it should be seen as a harmful practice.

In a course organized on ' Packaging Population Advocacy ' by Journalists in Accra, Ghana in 1998; Participants from Malawi, spoke of a practice, "where a young girl, on attainment of puberty and on the last day of her first menstruation is sent a 'fisi' or 'hyena'-an experienced man to formally introduce her to sex". It was also revealed that certain ethnic cultures within Malawi also encourage pre-marital sex as a way of proving the potency and fertility of adolescents. Zambia was also indicted in some of these unwholesome practices. Specifically, women are said to introduce foreign matters and herbs to dry up the vagina in readiness for what is referred to as ' dry sex '. For the woman according to the Zambian participants, the sexual act is usually a very painful experience. Among the Maasai of Kenya on the other hand, "the woman is regarded as a community property, as wife sharing is a common practice". Here husband does not have an exclusive right to his wife. More so, Maasai women have ways of keeping lovers

---

[125] Lucas Lukumbo 1998, Pp. 10.

outside matrimony. The ' Trokosi ' practice in some part of Ghana, is another typical case of subjugation of women reproductive and sexual health rights; the practice is such that, " young female virgins are sent to the shrine to atone for the crime committed by their forebears and such girls are forced to have sex with the priest."[126]

These cultural practices are not only harmful, but also undermine the reproductive rights of such women, to decide freely and responsibly, the number and spacing of their children and how to do so. It also includes the right to attain the highest standard of sexual and reproductive health and also the right to make decisions on discrimination, coercion and violence.[127]

Consequently, reproductive health as an embodiment of health whose components include family planning, maternal and child health, management of STD's, menopause and andropause; also include the management of cancers of the reproductive organs such as cervical, breast and prostate cancer, prevention and management of unsafe abortion, information and counselling on human sexuality, responsible sexual behaviour and responsible parenthood; particularly as it affects adolescents.[128]

---

[126] Nigerian Vanguard Newspaper 1998, Pp. 10.
[127] Henrietta Odoi-Agyarko 1998, Pp. 10.
[128] Ibid 1998, pp. 10.

5.0. Chapter five

5.1. Women Resistance and Complicity to Socio-Cultural and Legal arguments on Reproductive Health

It has been recorded in World demographic estimates that women accounts, for more than half of the global population. Yet the status of women continues to be substantially inferior to that of men (UN 1989) Worldwide, for example, women continue to have the highest rates of illiteracy, to earn significantly less money than men even when performing the same work, and to have fewer legal protection available to them for helping in resolving disputes. The small number of women worldwide who occupy important positions, of political or policy - making power is already well established.[129]

Certainly, the majority of women in developing countries are yet to realize the minimal economic objectives, legal protections, and the political aspirations that were sought as part of the International Decade of Women from 1975-1985. The reasons for lack of more substantial social progress for women over the past two decades are many but centre on several realities, such that;

• development efforts, in the main continue to be directed at improving the social and economic conditions of men in developing countries,

• the role of women as co-partners, let alone as leaders, in development has been grossly under estimated by the international development community and,

• the assistance strategies of the majority of international development organizations, intentionally or not, have functioned to perpetuate social and economic inequalities, which for countries have retarded the social progress of women.

It is in the realization of these perpetuated gender based inequalities which works to the detriment of women everywhere, that has propelled and imposed on women themselves the necessary burden to fight for the improvement of their status (rights). They were to discover that the best way to assert their rights is to defend and uphold it. This situation has given rise to women globally, to form organizations, associations, movements and to join issues with Non Governmental Organizations (NGOs) to fight for the legal protection of their rights; and one of such rights is the recent advocates for the "reproductive rights of the woman" and her access to safe abortion and reliable methods of contraception, and the legislation against female circumcision and other harmful traditional practices against women.[130]

However, the 1960s marked the rise of the Women's movement, of which reproductive rights is a fundamental corner stone. Some clamour for abortion

---

[129] Richard J. Estes 1992, 1-2
[130] Sue Armstrong 1991, Pp.42-44

rights for pregnant victims of rape or incest or when the mother's health is at risk. Medical technology has opened a window on the womb to sport possible birth defects and the baby's gender. Pregnancies are ended on the strength of a doctor's pessimistic prognosis. Women over 40 years of age may be anxious about deformities.[131]

In poverty striking land, many women who have limited access to contraception feel they cannot provide for more children. And stretching the definition of 'pro-choice' to its limits, some pregnant women choose to abort a foetus because they feel that the timing of the pregnancy is just not right or because they learn the sex of the unborn child and simply do not want it. In Nigeria, where abortion is illegal and the laws for its operation is still highly restrictive, women make up the strongest opposition to it. Surprisingly, men seem to be much more willing to accept the idea than most middle class women (Qualls, 1990). Thus, despite the existence of a motley of women organizations like the, National Council for Women Society (NCWS), Gender and Development Action (GADA), Women In Nigeria (WIN), International Women's Health Coalition (IWHC), Women's Right Project (WRP), Women Health Organization of Nigeria (WHON), Society for Women and AIDS in Africa-Nigerian chapter, Federation of International Women's Lawyers In Nigeria etc., their activities are still somewhat restrictive in the struggle for the reproductive rights of the woman, particularly as it affect the right of abortion and the adoption of contraception as a 'pro-choice' instrument and the legislation against female circumcision. This is because of the strong cultural or traditional beliefs and practices as it relates to the twin issue of abortion and contraception, and female circumcision.

Cross nationally, women from developed western countries such as United States of America, Britain, Australia, Germany, Wales, Scotland, Sweden etc, have been more aggressive, consistent and astute in their demand for reproductive rights of women. Specifically, in Australia, 'the Women Electoral Lobby (WEL)' represents the interests of all Australian women in maintaining their rights to choose. She has taken up a number of legal actions to protect the rights of the women in terms of abortion and contraceptives issues. While in the U.S.A, the California Abortion Rights Action League (CARAL) is an NGO with predominant women members that uses the political process to generate the full range of the reproductive rights to all women; that is, to support and protect, as a fundamental freedom a woman's right to make reproductive choices.

In Africa, the South African Women's movements seem to be in the forefront of the campaign for the legislation against female circumcision, and for a law in support of abortion, and the recognition of the woman's right to choose. In fact, the feminist wing of the African National Congress (ANC) is, the arrowhead, of the campaign. Some 'anti-abortion' feminist movements argue that the South

---

[131] Awake 1993, Pp.4.

African example is a peculiar case, against the background that the country has the highest cases of rape in world; and that with the number put at 52,000 and the predominance of the HIV infected persons. The situation is understood.[132] More so, it is the belief of such women's movement that the practice of female circumcision does not exist in most South African cultures.

While in Algeria, a predominantly Islamic state ruled by religious laws, the women rights activists, pointed out that a woman can only undergo abortion when or if certified or adjudged medically insane or she is known, to have been raped. According to the Women's Right President, the stigma attached to rape in Islamic society like Algeria effectively destroys women's life, and that their struggle for the amendment of the law to these categories of women only came to fruition in 1998 after a very long struggle. In her words, "this was a tremendous amendment to the abortion law after many years of traumatic experiences; because hundred of children born as a result of these attacks are subsequently abandoned."[133]

Today, the Centre for Reproductive Law and Policy (CRLP), an international Non Governmental Organization (NGO) now has its spread in most African countries (including Nigeria) dedicated to ensuring that all women have access to appropriate and freely chosen reproductive health services. Consequently, all women's reproductive rights movements in collaboration with the NGO work through the political process and through grassroots education and outreach programmes, developing strategies to promote policies that; (a) ensure all women the constitutionally protected right to choose to continue a pregnancy with access to quality pre-natal care or to obtain a safe, legal abortion; (b) ensure that women and men have access to quality sexuality education and voluntary contraceptive care in order to prevent unintended pregnancy; (c) ensure that these rights and the conditions necessary to exercise these rights are available to everyone without regards to race, ethnicity, colour, religion, age gender, degree or physical ability, national origin, sexual orientation, marital status, political affiliation, economic means, or educational status.[134]

5.2. Women's Movement and the Campaign for Reproductive Health Rights in Nigeria

Familial roles were traditionally the basis on which Nigerian women were organized within their villages and communities, particularly, around activities such as circumcision, childbirth and marriage rites. In fact, work groups formed the basis of women's rich associational history in pre-colonial times. Women

---

[132] 'Rape cases and the spread of HIV in South Africa', BBC news on Africa, broadcasted on November 29, 1999 at 18.00 GMT.
[133] 'Algeria authorises abortion for rape victims', BBC news on Africa, broadcasted on April 12, 1998 at 15.22 GMT.
[134] The California Abortion and Reproductive Rights Action League (CARAL)-'Promoting Reproductive Choices-The Choice Report' Fall 1999 Pp.1-8.

were also active in organizations established to protect their communities. These association's unquestionably provided women with necessary support and camaraderie. However, in keeping with the values that underlay tradition and religion, these activities tended to reinforce and reproduce the structures of patriarchy through which women were subordinated.

Most of these women movements and organization in Nigeria have tackled both the difficulties posed by the relics of traditional and cultural practices and also, fresh problems caused by the dynamics of modernization. Generally, rural women's group identified with traditional activities, such as initiations rites, which have declined in number and significance as cultural values and practices have gradually began to change. However, and most unfortunate, is that the majority of presently emerging women's organization meant to champion the cause of women's rights and to advance gender consciousness in society are located in principal urban centres. This problem is further compounded in the words of Sociologists Kisekka that, "it cannot, however, be accurately inferred that there is a women's movement in the country which is vociferously engaged in the exposure and challenge of gender inequality (and by extension, the reproductive health rights of women) in most of its ramifications. Rather, most women's associations have striven to operate cautiously within traditional gender boundaries articulating the theory of complimentary rather than competitive roles in gender relations."[135]

Again, the conflict among women's groups or association with regards to the term 'feminist orientation' has hindered their struggle for reproductive health rights and equality. Most of the women object to the term 'feminism' or 'feminist' orientations. Those objecting to the feminist label view it as Western terminology that should not be employed in Africa or Nigeria for that matter. It is the belief of these group of women that when "the African women demand equality, we are only asking for rights not to be tampered with, and the removal of laws that oppress and dehumanises women. We are not asking for equality with our husbands. We accept them as our bosses and heads of the family". This sort of assertion has helped men to exercise their masculine roles over women unknowingly to them. This is because African men see nothing wrong in their relationships with Western governments and institutions, but object to African women having relationships with these same institutions. These same institutions have made cases like female circumcision to thrive in practicing Urhobo, Isoko and Okpe ethnic groups in Nigeria. This is because, women's economic subordinate status renders them economically and socially dependent on their husbands and fathers in crucial decisions that affect their bodies, making it difficult for those of them who do not want to undergo the operation of female circumcision or keep an unwanted pregnancy to make independent decisions. Thus international and national women organizations are engaged in encouraging

---

[135] Mere Kisekka 1992, Pp. 51.

many young women to take up professional courses so that they will be economically independent and be able to take care of issues that demand independent actions without being made to depend on financial assistance from their husband and fathers.[136]

Thus, the notion that women are bounded together by a common history of oppression and a common struggle to achieve liberation does not hold true in Nigeria. There are secondary divisions in any social movement that create obstacle for the realization of group objectives, even within a single-sex movement like the women's movement.[137]

In Nigeria, these cleavages and divisions among women are based on religion, age, marital status, ethnic origin, educational level and social class. Tensions and conflicts within the women's movement have been based in part on differences over strategy and policy, and in part on leadership struggles. The Nigerian women movement cannot be faulted for not being a homogenous organized body. Rather, it consist of several groups, all of which are arguing in different, and at times conflicting, ways about matters affecting women based on differing perception of women's interests.

However, a fundamental question that emerges is whether the activities of the existing women movements, groups, associations and organizations are emancipatory, or subordinatory in their struggle. Thus, women's movement in Nigeria should realize that the issues of women's reproductive rights and choice, female circumcision, sexual harassment and violence, abortion and consciousness raising program in the broader discourse on women is incontrovertible.

Consequently, the combination of continuity and change in women's organizations suggests, however, that the question of whether Nigerian women are moving toward achieving emancipation or remain subordinated is not a simple one. While the women's movement is fluid and experience historical shifts in its class and urban-rural composition are evident, it is clear that winning over the rural women who form the back bone of the nation and the object of most of the reproductive health oppression is the key to its continuous progress.

5.3. The Genesis of Women Reproductive Health in Nigeria Population Policy

The relationship between Nigerian women and the state requires serious thoughts in this dimension. The 'woman question' is important because of the close attention or relationship it has to other issues such as gender relations, ethnicity, religion and national development. The issue of reproduction and reproductive health stand out. Though, women have enjoyed more attention in this aspect than

---

[136] Efua Dorkenoo 1995, Pp. 159.
[137] Amrita Basu 1995, Pp. 213.

men, it is clear that a good portion of this attention has not served women well. This is because it has been built on unfavourable gender relations and helps to perpetuate a range of subordinate relationships between men and women as well as serve the state interest.

The issue of women reproductive health in Nigeria population policy came to limelight in about the 1960s when the International Population establishment became interested in Africa's population growth rate. Even with this focus the Nigerian government resisted advice on the pressure over fertility control through the 1970s until about the mid-1980's. Before this time Nigerian physicians had for a long time been privately concerned about mortality rates and the health of the mother and children. However, the push from the West to link fertility to national development in Third World nations only made an impact as each African nation sank into an economic crisis. It was within this context, the Nigerian state made a turn around and constructed a National Population Policy in 1988 that was implemented in 1989. The summary of the policy include the under listed highlights,

- To reduce the percentage of women who bear more than four children by fifty percent by 1995 and by eighty percent in year 2000.
- To extend family planning service to fifty percent of women by 1995 and eighty percent in the year 2000.
- To reduce total fertility rate of women from over six (6) to four (4) in the year 2000.
- To reduce the population growth rate from 3.3 percent per annum to 2.5 by 1995 and 2.0 percent by the year 2000.
- To reduce Infant Mortality Rate (IMR) by 50 percent by 1990.
- To reduce the percentage of women who get married before 18 years by fifty percent in 1995 and eighty percent by the year 2000.
- To reduce pregnancy below 18 years and above 35 years by fifty percent by 1995 and ninety percent by the year 2000

In the pre-colonial era, because of the patrilineal / patrilocal extended family system, issues of reproductive health was overlooked. In fact, pregnancy and delivery is usually not thought of as 'work', But as Rothman points out, pregnancy is work, because in addition to the physical burden, all societies have behavioural expectations regarding it.[138]

The colonial era did not help matters. In fact, at this time, women suffered important set backs economically and politically, because of the gender dimension of the formation. In fact, women were particularly disenfranchised as the process of indirect rule rendered them invisible in the governing process and

---

[138] Barbara Katz Rothman 1989, Pp. 3-9.

challenged their decision- making roles in the economy. This contributed to the loss of their status.[139] All of these were carried over into independence, which made women to lose ground at the local, state and federal levels on issues to men. Once formed the male dominated state had the power to further construct gender relations in homes, community and beyond, after independence. This became an important input in constructing 'population problems' and programmes for fertility control. Except for a few issues such as abortion, the Nigerian government stayed out of the World population debate until the mid-1980s. So, despite her taking part in the signing of major international resolutions on women's health, thereafter, there was no commitment on her part to implement the resolutions back home. This has been the trend ever since with the plight of women's health.

The above situation has engendered the emergence of concerned women organizations, as well as non -governmental organizations and various other international agencies to embark on the constant trend of campaigns and awareness programmes for the improvement and inclusion of women's health and activities on major governmental health policy projects.

---

[139] Johnson-Odim and Mba 1997, Pp. 68.

6.0. Chapter six

6.1. The Nigerian Constitution and the Woman

The Nigerian constitution has failed to address and protect women from various forms of prejudices. The inbuilt prejudices in the 1979 and lately, in the 1999 constitution against females and the language in the document failed to emphasize the equality of every citizen. These inbuilt, prejudice violates their rights in the name of restrictive religious practices, customary and statutory laws.

Some female scholars argue, "the constitution which represents the basic law of the state must contain adequate provisions on matters regarding women, if they are to participate fully as citizens in a society which claims to operates the principles of democracy" They stressed that in Nigeria, laws have been deliberately misinterpreted and manipulated to suit the male ego. They also, contended that there ought to be legislative provisions as well as guidelines regulating rampant cases of girls-child marriage, contraception and religious practices which will give equal rights to both men and women.[140]

Complementing the above concern for women's right and the constitution, Donli, Hansine, in a paper titled, *Women, Fundamental Rights and Justice,* lamented the lack of protection, of the Nigerian woman from dehumanising customs and traditions such as female circumcision and widowhood which is predominant amongst the Bini and Igbo speaking ethnic groups in Nigeria. The problem of the widow in her view is often compounded by the suspicious attitude of the in-laws towards her as having a hand in the death of the husband. The outcome of this is the dehumanisation of the widow in the guise of proving her innocence by making her to cut her hair, sit on the flour for the period until the dead man was buried, as well as making the woman to drink from a concoction made from the bathed dead body of the late man etc.[141]

Sako, Rebecca on her part, indicted women for failing on their own to study the provisions in the constitution that affects them. In her words, "the problems affecting women and the society at large, is the ignorance of provisions of the constitution. According to her, the constitution contains the laws and rules that establish and regulate government activities. The constitution also contains rules and laws that impose or purports to impose rights and responsibilities on citizens, which are collectively called fundamental rights. A good citizen should know what the constitution says on what issues."[142]

Giwa-Osagie in his own paradigm on, *Women's Health in the 21st Century*, noted " ...that while women made more significant gains in the last century, they could not be said to have achieved much because of the socio-economic disadvantage

---

[140] J. Nasir, 'Women activists criticise constitution' in the Guardian online: www.ngrguardiannews.com, Sunday, January 30, 2000.
[141] ibid
[142] ibid.

in a male dominated world and their lack of mutual cooperation. He stressed that lack of access to health care and gender discrimination, which the Nigerian woman suffers, had resulted in a horrifying maternal mortality rate that is said to be one of the highest in the World. Furthermore, he pointed out that haemorrhage (excessive bleeding), infections (sepsis), hypertension disorders (eclampsia), prolonged obstructed labour and unsafe abortion constitute major preventable causes of maternal deaths in the country." He contended that maternal mortality in Nigeria was more than a health issue but also a human rights issue that must be addressed by the Nigerian constitution, and that solution to the problem of women's health lay in the provision of access to health care under a more humane legislative health environment.[143]

The United Nations (UN), in its 1999 annual report on Development and other related issues throughout the world revealed that, "the annual income from sexual exploitation of women and children worldwide is put at 7 billion dollars"[144] This is perhaps an indication that sexual exploitation is now a booming business. It however, emphasized a strict legislative interference to protect women and children's rights in this regards. Unfortunately, the Nigerian experience is a complicated one where resorts to cultural and religious references have been prominent in the debate for constitutional provisions to protect the rights of the woman.

6.2. The Nigerian Constitution on Abortion, Contraception and Female Circumcision

Globally, about 62 percent of the world people live in countries where induced abortion is permitted either for a wide range of reasons or without restriction as to any form of reasons. In contrast, about 25 percent of all people reside in nations where abortion is generally prohibited.[145]

However, in Nigeria where the constitution is not clear about it, the country's Criminal law specifically is emphatic about the restriction of abortion and the adoption of contraception. Under the Criminal Code, abortion can only be allowed to save the life of the pregnant woman. Thus, the law explicitly exempts from punishment, providers (qualified professional medical practitioners) or women who undergo abortions when the woman's life is in danger.

In the 'Laws of the Federation of Nigeria and Lagos' which was in force on the First day of June, 1958, chapter 42 of the Criminal Code, section 228 state "any

---

[143] Osato Giwa-Osagie, 'HIV/AIDS: Women more at Risk' on Vanguard online: www.vanguardngr.com, Thursday, January 27, 2000.

[144] Dickson Adeyanju, '$7b earned yearly on sexual exploitation of women' in Guardian online: www.ngrguardiannews.com, Sunday, September 19, 1999.

[145] Centre for Reproductive Law and Policy- A special rapporteur on violence against women issued a report in January 1999 entitled "Policies and practices that impacts women reproductive rights and contribute to causes or constitute violence against women" (E/CN.4/1999/68/add.4)

person who with intent to procure miscarriage of a woman whether she is or she is not with child, unlawfully administers her to take any poison or other noxious thing, or uses any force of any kind, or uses any other means whatever, is guilty of felony, and is liable to imprisonment for fourteen years". Also, section 229 of the same Criminal Code state, "any woman who with intent to procure her own miscarriage, whether she is or is not with child, unlawfully administers to herself poison or other noxious thing, or uses any force of any kind, or uses any such thing or means to be administered or used to her, is guilty of a felony, and is liable to imprisonment for seven years"

The above two quoted sections of the Criminal Code clearly state the implications for both the conductor of the action and the woman. They are both regarded as criminals for engaging in the acts as prescribed by the law. The Criminal Code went further to state in section 230 of the same chapter 42 that, "any person who unlawfully supplies to or procures for any person anything whatever, knowing that it is intended to be unlawfully used to procure the miscarriage of a woman, whether she is or is not with child, is guilty of a felony, and is liable to imprisonment for three years". However, these three sections clearly state that, "the offender can not be arrested without a warrant"

These provisions raised series of unanswered issues such as, 'will the health of the existing children in the family be a factor to take into account?' Also today, some jurisdictions think that even the health of the child to be born is a factor to be taken into account. Again, where the pregnancy came about as a result of felonious intercourse such as rape, incest etc., Should these not be good grounds for justifying termination of pregnancy? While these unanswered questions still poses as the most contentious issues between the pro and anti advocates of legalization of abortion, section 232 of the Penal Code Law, Cap 89 laws of Northern Nigeria 1963, clearly sums up the Nigeria legal position as, "whoever voluntarily causes a woman with child to miscarry shall, if such miscarriage be not caused in good faith for the purpose of saving the life of the woman, be punished with imprisonment for a term which may extend to fourteen years or with fine or with both". It should be noted that the Penal Code is a slight modification of the Criminal Codes Chapter 42, Sections 228, 229, and 230; because of its emphasis on a proven case that the woman must be certified to have been with child before she perpetuated the act. However, the laws of the Federal Republic of Nigeria, surpasses that of any regional parts of its federation.

What should be noted therefore, is that the laws of Nigeria is still very emphatic on the illegality of abortion and the procurement of contraception for the same. In the same vein, aiding and abetting in the act itself also constitutes a punishable crime under the law.

On the issue of female circumcision the constitution does not say anything about it. In fact, it is silent with regards to that. That is a clear allusion to the fact that the constitution with regards to reproductive health of women is still inadequate and needs some basic amendments in line with series of conferences resolutions and the United Nations (UN) resolution on such culturally harmful practices on the health of the woman.

7.0. Chapter Seven

7.1. Theoretical Framework

There are several existing Sociological theories that explain social change in society. The focus of these theories, are on the progress, stability, growth, better life, freedom and rights of the individual and the overall development of society. Some of such theories include, Evolution, Diffusion, Structural Functionalism, Modernization, and Conflict theories. However, most of the mentioned theories lack in adequacy of assumptions and explanations of the research interest under study and thus, undermine the basis for their adoption in this research study.

Consequently, this study adopt the Structural Functional, Conflict and Modernization theoretical frame works for its explanation because the three accommodated and made provisions for the neglect inherent in the other theories. Specifically, the Conflict theory, understand the polemic and power play involved in advocating legislation on abortion and against female circumcision. On its part the Modernization theory, explains the fundamental basis for the need for such legislations; while the Structural Functionalist argue on the need for the perpetuation of certain cultural practices on basis of their functionality for the maintenance of social order in the existing societies. In this case, the issue on the legislation against abortion, and the continuation of female circumcision. The details of the individual theories are discussed underneath.

7.2. The Functionalist Theory

This perspective emphasizes functional integration and social structure in society. It was made popular by Parsons, Talcott and Robert K. Merton. Most of their ideas were drawn from Durkheim and Weber.[146]

The functionalist, are more concerned with the functions of various phenomena than with trying to ascertain the 'real nature' of the phenomena. Thus, they are of the philosophy which, in recognizing the values set up by every society to guide its own life, lays stress on the dignity inherent in everybody, of custom, and on the need for tolerance of conventions though they may differ from ones own. To them, all aspects of cultures in any society play a valid and functional role to the stability of that society. They looked at the society as an organism with structure or component parts, each of these parts acting together to maintain the whole. Stability (social order) was highly emphasized.

The main thrust of this theory, is that a change in any part of society's units is seen as leading to a certain degree of imbalance, which in turn result in changes in other parts of the system and a total re-organization of the system to an equilibrium state. They argue on this basis, 'the right of man to live in terms of their own tradition'.

---

[146] Gordon Marshall 1998, Pp.248

More so, the functionalist postulates the indispensability of the structural units or functions in social system by neglecting the possibility of the functional substitutes or of the use of alternative units to attain the goals of society.[147]

Functionalist, further argue that any cultural practice must be functional or it will disappear before long. That is, it must somehow, contribute to the survival of the society. To them, many cultural functions are not manifest but latent. In fact, Merton illustrates the basic point that a function may be manifest (that is, obvious or intended) or latent (that is, hidden or unintended).

On this basis, those who antagonize the legislation on the liberalization of abortion, and advocate for the continuation of female circumcision hinge their argument. For such individuals, banning abortion or allowing a law as it is, as well as continuing the practice of female circumcision helps to sustain the moral basis of society. For instance, they opined that allowing abortion to be liberalized would not only increase the rate of sexual promiscuity, but also, lead to moral decadence in the society. The same moral thesis has been put forward as argument for the sustenance of female circumcision as well as the enhancement of fertility, neatness, respect, initiation to womanhood etc. All of these to them help not only to aid social integration but social solidarity in the society.

Functionalists thus, argue that those calling for legislation for the liberalization of abortion and against female circumcision are 'iconoclasts' whose views are not part of the institution which direct social action; and that if you study the background of these people, you will find out that their ideas are borne out of particular experiences and not their objective views. Mary Douglas holds that such iconoclastic views tend to hinder classifications, thus they should be segregated, isolated, separated and considered anomalies.[148]

The functionalist, also, believe that the modernization theorists have failed to look into the genetic basis that informed the practice of female circumcision in many culture areas before attacking it. They accused the modernist of focusing on the manifest reasons (that is, the health implications); and neglecting the latent reasons (that is, the genetic explanations) for the practice before engaging in the campaign for its discontinuation.

Further more, they are of the view that the modernization theory only addresses the moral aspect of female circumcision without discussing the technological aspect for the medicalization of the process that makes it physically and physiologically dangerous to the health of the woman. To them rather than challenge social facts and reduce it to individualism, they should look at female circumcision as a 'collective phenomena' not reducible to the individual actor or psyche, and help to refine the culture of the practice by improving the technological process for the sake of morality.

---

[147] Onigu Otite and William Ogionwon 1981, Pp. 21.
[148] Mary Douglas 1966, Pp. 116.

7.3. The Modernization Theory

Modernization theorists view the functionalist approach to the study of social phenomena as too culturally relativistic. It is important for this researcher to paraphrase the ideas of Robert Redfield in this context, "…it is not arguable against the obvious fact that truths (institutions, values) may be regarded as relative to time, place and particular culture. But it should be asserted that acceptance of functionality of cultural units does not necessitate rejections of all value commitments."[149] Redfield's assertion has immense practical significance to this study, because he points to the dangers, as well as to the logical fallacies, of those who would say, for example, "since everything is right (functional) in terms of its own logic, I cannot condemn the excesses of totalitarianism." As Redfield shows, science itself would cease to exist if such an attitude were carried to its logical conclusion.

The modernization theory was dominant amongst Sociologists and Economists in the 1950s. The proponents include, Wilbert Moore, Levi Straus, Alex Inkeles, Michael Todaro, and Walt Whitman Rostow. It focused on the total transformation of tradition and pre-modern into the type of technology associated with social organizations that characterize the advanced economically prosperous and relatively stable nations, of the western world.[150]

From the socio-economic perspective, modernization theory, views economic development as dependent on cultural attitudes. Thus, the theory holds that development depends on certain pre-requisites, especially positive cultural attitudes towards progress and willingness to change.

Consequently, much attention was focused on identifying the social and cultural conditions that would be required for developing nations to 'take off' towards positive growth and development.[151] That is, developing countries (poor countries), it was thought, were missing crucial cultural traits such as self-discipline, rationality, willingness to change, devotion to hard work etc. that Max Weber attributed to the protestant reformation.

Socio-culturally, modernization theorists view modernity and tradition as polar opposites. For them, society can only modernize when they must have overcome their traditionalism. They hold the views that underdevelopment is an original state from which all societies start in relation to the goal of development and change. In fact, the most important contribution of modernization theory is its emphasis on culture, on the ideas and attitudes that promotes innovation.[152] Therefore, for a significant structural change to take place in any society, concomitant transformations in attitudes, institutions and ideologies are often

---

[149] Robert Redfield 1960, Pp. 32.
[150] Michael P. Todaro 1982, Pp.352
[151] Walt Whitman Rostow 1952, Pp.1-4
[152] Alex Inkeles 1983, Pp. 18

necessary. Obvious examples of these transformations include the general urbanization process and the adoption of the ideals, attitudes and institutions of what has come to be known as modernization.[153]

Consequent on the above, the modernization advocates argue that, the continued growth in the total size of the human population in Nigeria due to the sharp increase in the birth rate after the civil war in 1970 should be viewed with grave concern. The average Nigerian woman has six children. While the emphasis, on agrarian activities has declined drastically, with diversion to technological and industrial activities. The need for more children has become highly unnecessary. Thus, with the rapid increasing urbanization (which create high unemployment, sub-standard housing, sewage and waste disposal problems and rising crimes); coupled with food shortages, environmental degradation, poor economy, continuous corruption has become the bane of the average individual, family and community in Nigeria. All these obvious, social, cultural, economic and environmental problems have been compounded by the lack of adequate legal mechanism to reduce the birth rate, particularly through the legalization or liberalization of abortion and access to contraceptives. As a result, women (adolescent females in particular) resort to illegal, induced and unsafe abortions to expel unwanted pregnancies. Whereas, the dangers associated with such act are immeasurable and colossal.

Also, the continuous practice of female circumcision in the name of culture, tradition, and religion, is viewed by modernization theorists as inimical to the health of the girl child. In effect, to modernization theorists, it affects the positive development of society if she must rely, on the contribution of women to the socio-economic development of society.

In this context, Modernization theorists view Functionalists in terms of legislation on abortion and against female circumcision, as being blurred by the factual realities of the necessities for such laws. For modernist, "certain cultural premises may become totally out of accord with a new factual situation. People (leader) may recognize this and reject the old ways in theory. Yet their emotional loyalty continues in the face of reason because of intimate conditioning of early childhood or the concept of what is called tradition or culture.[154]

Contextually, the modernization theory help to understand and evaluate the 'modern Nigerian individual mind' in terms of its attitudes as it relates to the embodiments of such ideals as efficiency, diligence, frugality, honesty, rationality, change, orientation, integrity, self-reliance, co-operation and willingness to take a long and thorough view of change. In other words, to them, "…what underdeveloped nations need is not only a scientific and technological

---

[153] Michael P. Todaro 1982, Pp. 352-360.
[154] Clyde Kluchhohn 1960, Pp. 74

society, which employs new techniques whether on the farm, in the factory, or in transport, but also, follows modern thinking."[155]

To modernization theorists, the quest for rationality implies that opinions about public and social policies should be logically valid inferences which are rooted as deeply as possible in knowledge of relevant facts; and an enlightened government could mobilize poplar support needed to overcome the inhibiting and often divisive forces of sectionalism and traditionalism in a common quest for wide spread material and social progress, particularly as it has to do in this instance with adolescent females reproductive health.

Finally, Modernization advocates, in reacting to the views of functionalist that, female circumcision and the law against the liberalization of abortion are social facts, argued that 'since society is changing; thoughts, perceptions, feelings are equally flowing in the direction of re-examining, re-evaluating, and re-viewing social facts. Consequently, individuals, institutions and disciplines may not be held responsible for this flaw (if it is). Since, it is manifestly justified that female circumcision does a lot of danger to the health of the woman, as well as induced and illegal abortion, the position of advocates for legislation against female circumcision and liberalization of abortion cannot, but be taken very seriously and sustained.

7.4. The Conflict Theory

This theory is predicated on the fundamental premise that at all level of social life, there exist, a pronounced measure of conflict. Conflict theory emphasizes the importance of interests over norms and values, and the way in which the pursuit of interests generated various types of conflict as normal aspects of social life, rather than abnormal or dysfunctional occurrences.[156] The theory has as its main thrust the proposition that, there is nothing like 'harmonious society' or a society that is intrigue free. Consequently for there, to be a progressive change, in the structure of society, there are bound to be dissenting and conflicting ideas in strict competition for dominance. The main proponents of conflict theory include, Karl Marx, Friedrich Engels, Ralf Dahrendorf, and John Rex.

While positing the inevitability of conflict in all existing social relationships, Karl Marx (1818-1883), pointed out that "...the view that all societies were progressing towards a state of peace and harmony, is utopian". He further explained that this is because, "even the implementation of what are taken as commonly defined good and progressive policies often lead to social conflict". This position is clearly manifested in this case. For instance, the induced decline in infant mortality rate raised the birth rate in most underdeveloped countries,

---

[155] Jawaharlal Nehru, 'Strategy of the third Plan.' In *Problems in the Third Plan: a critical miscellany*; Government of India; Ministry of Information and Broadcasting, 1961, Pp. 46
[156] Gordon Marshall 1998, Pp. 108.

which has in turn encouraged certain members in these countries to press for birth control techniques. Such efforts at birth control have in their own turn involved conflicts with traditional and religious institutions.[157] In other words, only rarely can a particular decision be taken to represent the 'general will' of a population and thus, most societies have institutionalised techniques by which the interest or views of certain sections of the population may be legitimately overridden.

But classical and contemporary Conflict theorists aggregate their theses on conflict on the following common premises:

• That all existing societies are made up of social beings,

• That these social beings are often from different socio-cultural, economic, political, and biological background;

• That as a consequence, there exist peculiarities among individuals, groups, and societies, as a result of their different beliefs, practices, values and culture,

• That since human beings must engage in social relationships, and most of these social relationships are often in pursuit of common interests, there are bound to be conflict of ideas, conceptions, values, cultures, beliefs and practices in the process of harmonizing these divergent differences and creating social order in the social structure;

• That the above situation always result in conflict between individuals; individuals and groups; groups and groups; groups and the institutional establishments in an attempt for the dominant accepted position to emerge.[158]

• On the basis of these assumptions, the Conflict theoretical framework is relevant to the research under study. More so, considering the fact that Nigeria is a multi ethnic, multi-cultural and multi-religious entity, the idea to legislate on abortion and against female circumcision was bound to evoke a lot of controversy, especially as it affects women in general and the adolescent females in particular, who are often regarded as the tender and most delicate category of any country's population.

On the basis of conflict theoretical analysis, the antagonists of liberalization of abortion and legislation against female circumcision hinge their opinion on the fact that, the idea is a foreign approach to the concept of 'family', that runs contrary to the African culture. According to them the African culture is that which respects the life of the unborn child since they are regarded as the wealth of tomorrow. To them abortion, is against the traditional beliefs and practices of the people, as killing under whatever guise is regarded as a cultural taboo. Also, to them the need for the beautification and initiation of the girl child into

---

[157] Onigu Otite and William Ogionwon 1981, Pp. 364.
[158] Avineri Shlomo 1968, Pp.3-4 and James A. Schellenberg 1996, Pp. 1-2.

womanhood, and the need also to enhance fertility respectively, are strong reasons for the continuous perpetuation of female circumcision. Thus, female circumcision to them is a symbol of African woman that is deeply rooted in the tradition and culture of the people.

Wolf-Dieter Just (1982), argued from what he termed the sociological evaluations of policies. He argued, that, "decisions and policies taken outside the circumstances of the people is the strongest cause of cultural alienation."[159] He also asserted that people ought to determine themselves and what they make of their world, otherwise, their human dignity is offended and the product of their culture made impossible. Others argue that, "any policy that is considered reasonable should emphasize the socio-cultural preferences of a people which determined their welfare."[160]

On the contrary, protagonists of liberalization of abortion and legislation against female circumcision found their arguments on the fact that, both processes are not really new to the socio-cultural and traditional practices of many ethnic groups in Nigerian. They further argued, that since man learned how to reproduce, there has been an eternal question of unwanted reproduction; and that the contemporary increase in modern society of unwanted, and unsafe abortions that are clandestinely perpetuated has spelt out more catastrophe than the preaching of morality of culture to facade infanticides. They further hold that women from Itsekiri, Benue and Akwa-Ibom speaking ethnic groups in Nigeria are culturally not circumcised and nothing happens, and that this empirical evidence should help to render all forms of cultural and traditional explanations for the sustenance of female circumcision in practicing areas a nullity.

In the light of the above, the Conflict theoretical framework highlights the divergent dimension of conflicts in the research under study:

• Gender specific conflict; that is the conflict between female protagonists for the legislation on the liberalization of abortion and legislation against female circumcision; and the male antagonists;

• Gender like conflicts; that is the conflicts among women, as well as among men in the light of the above;

• Conflict between women and the institutional establishments in term of advocating for their reproductive health and sexual rights;

• Conflicts between all individuals irrespective of sex, age and class, who are in support of the liberalization of abortion and the legislation against female circumcision, and the Nigerian government;

---

[159] Just Wolf-Dieter 1982, Pp. 40.
[160] D. T. Ellwood 1989, Pp. 6.

• Conflicts between functionalist (in this case traditionalists and conservatives) and modernization advocates in respect of the legislation on the issues of abortion and female circumcision.

Thus, as often happen when rapid social change occurs, the movement always generates resistance, and counter movements. In effect, the Conflict theory enables one to understand the socio-cultural dynamics of the existing social relations among the people as it relates to their reproductive health behaviour in terms of their knowledge, awareness, perception and practices of sex related issues; particularly as it centres on the issues of abortion and female circumcision amongst adolescent females in Nigeria.

8.0. Chapter eight

8.1. Research Methodology

Nigeria, apart from being the most populous in the sub-Saharan Africa, is also one of the largest in the sub-continent. The country is characterized by ethnic groups of different cultural patterns. Thus, in a study of this nature, the area of study was limited to two local government areas, the Sapele and Ethiope-East local government areas respectively, of Delta state. These local government areas share similar characteristics in terms of their cosmopolitan nature that make both a home to a number of ethnic communities. They both also, have a similar level of development, when measured in terms of infrastructural facilities and other socio-economic indices- education, income, housing, occupation etc.

8.2. Data Collection Techniques

This study is a qualitative research, and data was collected through the following qualitative methods,

• Focus group discussions, and

• Personal interviews (including case study)

Secondary sources of data collections like documentary evidence, where available was also, used to compliment respondents views. Since the major objective of this research is to understand, 'the legislation and socio-cultural impediments to abortion and against female circumcision', particularly with respect to adolescents females reproductive health; most of the questions because of their sensitivity were largely confined to adolescents. When adults were included, their views and results are presented accordingly to make for easy comprehension and necessary comparison.

The questions used as guides for the focussed group discussions and personal interviews (including case studies) was designed in the standard of the 'National Survey on Reproductive Health' by the Planned Parenthood Federation of America (PPFA) on adolescents sexuality and the World Health Organization (WHO) standard as adopted in the study of Reproductive Health Communication in Kenya (August-September, 1994)

The questions included discussions on personal information relating to family background, educational attainment, religious beliefs, age, occupation, relationship with others, etc. Then the research questions ranged from sexuality education, sex behaviour, pregnancy and abortion, female circumcision; knowledge, attitude, and practice of reproductive health services and advocacy, particularly with regards to abortion and female circumcision; federal and state legislations on both issues and personal views on reproductive and sexual health issues. In other words, personal views on reproductive and sexual issues were raised and discussed in focused group discussions, personal interviews and case studies sessions.

The data was collected during my fieldwork that spanned two summer-time frames between August 30 and November 20, 2000 and between September 31 and October 31, 2001 respectively, in Nigeria. During the periods, a total of four focus group discussion sessions was conducted with numbers of participants ranging between five and seven persons per session. While seventeen concrete personal interviews was concluded (including case study).

The total number of participants or respondents from the three categories of data collection source was forty- four. This number was made up of seventeen males and twenty-seven females.

The focus group discussion was held among homogenous groups, with the exception of the adult category that was heterogeneous in composition. The participants from the adolescent female bracket were drawn from three target groups namely:

- Adolescent females in schools (unmarried)

- Adolescent female not in school (married)

- Adolescent females not in school (unmarried)

Focus group discussion was also, conducted separately for other categories of respondents. These include, adolescent males as well as older and experienced adults (males and females). The purpose for this was to have a holistic view of the subject under research and to provide for an adequate scientific explanation of the findings. More so, it helped this researcher to make a reliable analysis of the views of all participants and established a trend in the findings. The homogeneous categorization of the adolescent focused group discussions also made for a sense of belonging and freedom of participation in discussions.

Contacts with all participants in the focused group was established by my research assistants; (a male), who work as a principal health officer, at the Primary health Centre; Amukpe- Sapele; and the other a female who is a senior mid-wife at the Family Planning Unit, in the ante-natal section of the Central Hospital, Sapele. By virtue of their professions and job, they (research assistants) both have constant contacts with schools, individuals, traditional and orthodox medical practitioners and other public institutions to discuss health matters that borders on restricted health issues. More so, they are seen as credible and trusted. Consequently, there was, not much of hitches in assembling the participants of the various categories, after initial personal attempts had failed.

Notable, was that adolescents who were not in school were drawn from within established household dwelling units, in line with the Primary Health Care listing in the area (omitting those who due to economic conditions had no fixed address)

Because, of the significance of the research to health matters. All the focus group discussions were held at the premises of the Primary Health Centre, at Amukpe,

Sapele. All participants found it convenient. Most of the discussions lasted for between two to three hours, while some of the sessions held for more than once.

The personal interviews were conducted in private homes and premises of respondents according to their wishes. The orthodox medical experts in this category, I had already known in a personal and working capacity; so there was no much of problems in initiating the contacts with them. The unorthodox expert health providers were introduced to me by their clients, most of whom are my neighbours and close family friends. So in all of the cases, the issue of trust and the need to ensure their anonymity was the watchword. The interviews lasted for a minimum of one hour and thirty minutes in each session.

The two case studies were identified during the focus group discussion. One was a victim of abortion and female circumcision combined. While the other one was not circumcised but a victim of abortion. The interview with them later took place at their individual private homes; and the interviews lasted for about one hour and thirty minutes each.

The language of discussion and interview was both English, and indigenous language (Okpe and Urhobo) as the context dictated. This was to enhance communication, understanding, reliability, flow and retrieval of data collected in situations where the respondents were illiterates or 'not too schooled'. Most of the English was 'pidgin' (that is, a form of corrupted English language), that is understood by every body in one form or the other.

In most of the sessions, I was the facilitator, assisted effectively by my trained co-assistants where necessary. Most of the focus group and interview sessions (including case studies) were taped and video recorded. But the orthodox medical experts and legislators opted to be off the records, on the ground of 'ethics' of their profession that does not allow such 'publicity' and also the cultural sensitivity of the issues discussed.

In all of the sessions, snacks was served to relax participants and create a spirit of oneness and togetherness; and also, gifts such as Condoms was distributed by this researcher to all participants as a way of enlightenment on the need for follow- up action as the research progressed.

In addition to the above, secondary data was extracted from literatures on reproductive health, particularly, on abortion, female circumcision, HIV/AIDS and other sexual behaviours of adolescents.

8.3. Data Analysis Techniques

Since, this research is qualitative, the analysis also adopted a qualitative and descriptive form, with a few emphasis on quantitative analysis to illuminate it where necessary.

The first step of the data analysis took a verbatim transcription and translation, as well as documentation of all recorded tapes (both cassettes and video tapes). The transcriptions included notes on sudden out bursts, hesitations, silence, enthusiasm and other indicators, which provided understanding of what transpired during the sessions.

From the transcribed records of each session, I was able to extract relevant information to the objective of the study. The verbatim transcription of the focussed group and interview sessions (including case study) was analysed sequentially using an aspect of logic of the 'objective hermeneutic' technique of text interpretation. I built a general picture on maximum and minimum views of respondents, without neglecting some of the findings that were specific. In fact, the challenge of this approach is that it does not only ensure that it is necessary for the researcher to identify the objective structural meanings and explanations of social phenomena, but it also, helped in highlighting the subjective structural meanings and explanations of social phenomena.[161] That is what Robert Merton referred to as the latent and manifest variables in the explanation of social phenomena.[162] It is in this context that social phenomena could be understood in a holistic sense.

Again, descriptive analysis was also, used to reveal the variability of views, opinions etc. among all the groups and participants in the study. Also, a simple cross tabulation analysis was drawn to establish socio-economic characteristics of all participants especially among the adolescents.

Finally, the end product of the analysis intends to provide an input into the action oriented, program by reflecting the feelings and aspirations of the adolescent females on the issue studied.

---

[161] Günter Burkart 1983, Pp. 24-48.
[162] Robert K. Merton 1960, Pp.22

9.0. Chapter nine

9.1. Ethnography of Nigeria

Nigeria is located in West Africa. The geographic coordinates lies between 10 °°
N and 8 °° E. She shares common borders with the Niger Republic in the North,
Cameroon and the Republic of Chad in the East, the republic of Benin in the
West and the Atlantic Ocean in the South.

Nigeria occupies a total landmass of 923,770 square kilometres, which is about
356,700 miles. About 910,770 square kilometres of the total land mass is made
up of solid land, while the remaining 13,000 square kilometres is occupied by
water. The total Land boundaries, is made up of about 4047 kilometres (2514
miles), while the Coastline occupies about 853 kilometres (530 miles).

According to the 1993 population estimates, about 9570 square kilometres is
made up of irrigated land. While land use is fragmented as follows,

• Arable land - 33 %

• Permanent Crops-3 %

• Permanent Pastures - 44 %

• Forests and Woodland - 12 %

• Others - 8 %

In climatic terms, Nigeria is located between the equator and the tropic of cancer.
This accounts for its hotness for most part of the year. Specifically, there are two
main types of temperatures regions. The tropical region in the South- with
temperatures usually at around 90°F and the sub-tropical regions in the North-
with temperature ranges between 60°F and 100°F. The temperatures are often
measured in Centigrade.

Nigeria has two main climatic seasons known as the Rainy and Dry seasons. The
rainy season often last between the months of May and September in the
Northern part of the country, and about the month of March and November in the
Southern part of the country.

On the other hand, the Dry season, often last during the remaining part of the
year. It is a period of very minimal rains. However, in the southern part of
Nigeria, there is also, a period around December till January called the
Harmattan season, during which the climate gets cold and dry. The wind that
causes this intermediate climate to occur in the South is referred to as the North -
East trade wind. It is often accompanied with a lot of dry wind. While the wind
that causes rain is referred to as the South-West Monsoon wind.

Nigeria has two major rivers, which flows through it; namely; the river Niger and
river Benue. However, the end region where the river Niger, meets the Ocean is
commonly referred to as 'Delta'. In spite, of these major rivers, there are other

smaller ones like, Rivers, Anambra, Cross-Rivers, Ethiope, Gongola, Hadejia, Kaduna, Katsinsa-Al, Kamadugu, Ogun, Osun, Owena, Osse, Sokoto, Yobe, Zamfara, Ethiope.

9.1.1. Demography

The issue of the exact number of people that inhabit Nigeria has been a source of controversy not only amongst the people themselves but also, with estimates that are computed by external and reputable international organizations like the United Nations (UN), World Bank, International Monetary Fund (IMF), Common Wealth etc. In fact, as it is clearly summarized by Chris Ugokwe, who was the immediate past chairman of the Nigeria Population Commission in 1998, "Population statistics have long been subject to dispute in Nigeria as the figures are used to determine some areas of state fund allocations". In spite, of these controversies the last official census of Nigeria held in 1991, put her population at 88 million. The same census figures put the annual growth rate of the population at 2.83 per cent. However, recent estimates from other sources put the Nigerian population at 113,828,587 million (July 1999). While the Criminal Investigation Agency (CIA) world fact book put the population at 101,232,251 (July 1995), and the annual population growth rate was put at 3.16 per cent.

Despite, these estimates, the issue that is not in contention is that Nigeria remains the most populous black, country in Africa, and the ratio between the male and female population seem to be almost equal.

9.1.2. People and Language

Just like the large number of people, so is the existing number of languages. Nigeria has more than 350 existing ethnic groups (by implication the same number of languages). However, only three (3) of the major ethnic groups languages known as; Yoruba (west), Ibo (east), and Hausa (north), are adopted as officially spoken along side the English language (official language) for business, economic, social and political transactions in the country. This situation has resulted in the cries of marginalisation by minority ethnic groups in the country. This has become a major problem in Nigeria today as a political configuration.

9.1.3. Polity

Nigeria operates a three (3) tier, system of government namely; the Federal, State, and Local governments respectively. Nigeria as a country attained independence in the year October 1st, 1960. Today, she is made up of thirty-six (36) states with the federal capital located centrally at Abuja (see Appendix V). Presently, Nigeria has transited from a military regime to civilian democracy on May 29, 1999. That makes it her fourth democratic experiment after series of military interventions since independence.

The form of government is the presidential federalism; made up of the Executive, Legislature and Judiciary. The executive organ of government is headed by, the president assisted by his vice-president and council of ministers. While the National Assembly, is bi-cameral in nature. It has the Senate (as the upper house), and the House of Representatives (as the lower house). They are both responsible for the enactment of laws that governs the federation. While the Senate is made up of equal numbers of representatives (3 members each) elected from each of the 36 states of the federation and one (1) from the federal capital territory (Abuja); the house of representatives are elected on the basis of the existing numbers of local governments areas in each state delineated into constituencies. In all, the Senate is made up of a total of 109 members (i.e. including a member representing the federal capital territory, Abuja); and the house of representative is made up of a total of 360 members.

The Judiciary interprets laws. It is constituted by the Chief Justice of the federation as the head, assisted by other appointed Judges in the federal Supreme Court, federal court of appeal, high courts, magistrate courts etc.

At the state levels the governors are the chief executives with their deputies and a council commissioners as effective assistants and political heads of ministries. There is a unicameral legislature in place with the responsibility to enact laws for the state, and the state judiciary saddled with the responsible of interpreting the laws.

 The third tier of government-known as the local government are headed by local government chairmen assisted by elected deputies and a constituted legislative house to run the business of governance at the grass root level. The country is divided into about 774 local governments areas. The funds for the running of the local government administration, is allocated by, the federal government with strict regulation and monitoring by the state governments.

In all of the three tiers system of governance, the 1979 constitution which was reviewed in 1999 by the military government and still under series of contention by the current civilian democratic dispensation serves as the effective guide (for now) of the actions and activities of those entrusted with administration. Notably is the fact, that the federal powers, prevails in any case of conflict of functions / responsibilities between the states and the federal.

9.1.4. Economy

Nigeria is not only vast in human resources but also, in economic resources. She is endowed with immense natural resources namely; petroleum, tin, iron ore, coal, limestone, zinc, lead, natural gas etc. In the agricultural sphere, she is blessed with products like, cotton, groundnuts, rubber, cocoa, rice, millet sorghum; animal resources like, cattle, goats, sheep, etc. However, she is presently mono-cultural in her economic activities by solely depending on oil. In fact, she ears more than 95 percent of her external earnings from oil to the neglect, of the other sectors especially agriculture. The form of agricultural practice is very subsistence, with more women engaged in it than men. Also, the agricultural sector suffers periodic natural hazards, such as periodic droughts, soil degradation, rapid deforestation, desertification, etc. all of these severely affect marginal agricultural activities in the country. Subsequently, the largely subsistence agricultural sector has failed to keep up with the rapid population growth. Now, Nigeria, which was once a large net exporter of food, must import food to sustain her large population.

Again, the insensitivity of both past military and civilian administrations, to diversify the Nigerian economy away from over dependence on the capital intensive oil sector which provides 30 percent of the Gross Domestic Product (GDP), and 95 percent f the foreign exchange earnings and about 80 percent of the budgetary revenues has led to the underdevelopment of the agricultural sector and other forms of small scale businesses. Consequently, Nigeria economy has suffered losses to multi-billion dollar tone in the agricultural sector and unbalanced terms of trade.

In spite, of these complexities most developed countries have taken advantage of the buoyant economic resources of Nigeria to establish both industrial and commercial business enterprises and companies in it.

9.1.5. Social Organization

Kinship formed the very basis of social organization in many ethnic groups in Nigeria. Kinship is regarded both as biological and socio-cultural phenomenon. Marriage and families are the key institutions in the creation of kinship ties among these ethnic groups especially among the Urhobo, Okpe and Isoko people. The family is regarded as a typical kinship unit and it provides the individual with the first and basic unit with which to identify. Consequently, kinship creates the most important condition for a strong social bond amongst the people. Here, the individual depends largely on relatives in his early socialization, and also, on them for major assistance during crisis periods.

The social organization system of many ethnic communities is paternally centred. Strictly, social organization in many ethnic groups is mainly a process whereby a male is head of the family, as well as the spiritual head. Women are mainly meant to perform subordinate roles in many of these ethnic groups. She is meant to be seen and not heard, to be assistants and not dominant in matters that are strictly socio-cultural. However, they are few women in many of these same ethnic groups like the men who hold certain political positions and help in the social and cultural organization of their communities. These women in power must have attained certain age and experienced or struck menopause (no more experiencing menstruation), and must have satisfied certain rite of passage requirement like going through the ritual of female circumcision. Such women are found in many Urhobo, Okpe, Isoko and Bini ethnic groups in Nigeria.

Consequently, emphasis on human development is more male centred than female. This account today, for the very wide disparity in inequality between women and men in education, economic, political, and social positions in both ethnic and Nigeria social and political structures. However, this trend is gradually changing with more awareness on the part of women in particular and society in general.

The issue of religion has unfortunately not helped matters. Though, the Nigerian society recognizes and practices multiple religious activities for a very long time ago -Traditional, Christian and Islamic etc. worships. All of these religions have been used to support the argument for the subordination of women in the social organization of the society. The northern part of Nigeria (19 states) is predominantly made up of Islamic religious followers, while all the states (17states) in the southern part of Nigeria are predominantly made up of Christian population. In fact, about 12 states in the Northern part of Nigeria apart from the moderate ones like, Plateau, Kogi, states have adopted full fledge Sharia rule making the state of women more precarious than ever, since separation has been adopted in the use of many public facilities between men and women. However, relatively women still enjoy some sanity in the south because of the liberal laws that are not tied strictly to the Christian religion.

Today, over fifty percent of the people are Moslems, forty percent Christians, and the remaining ten percents claims to be traditional religious worshippers and other forms of religions. Although, the above statistics has been a subject of controversy as to which of the religious faithful are more in number.[163]

Thus, social organization among many ethnic groups in Nigeria, make the individual not to live all his life in the kinship unit or the family alone, but also, to belong to the wider society and interact and share responses with people outside the family unit. In this structure, the family is therefore, regarded as a mediating unit between the individual and the wider social organization by training and preparing him for the assumption of positions and roles in the wider society. Consequently, the individual is protected at two different levels -the family and, the society.

9.2. Brief ethnographic account of Specific Research Areas

9.2.1. Sapele and Ethiope-East Local Government Areas

In writing this brief ethnography of both local government areas. This researcher strongly adopted a style of non- separation, since both local governments areas are proportionately similar by their socio-cultural, economic, and political

---

[163] John Chukwuemeka Aghadiuno, 'Religion in Nigeria'
www.aghadiuno.atfreeweb.com/religion, updated and accessed on 22.03.2001

characteristics. Also, they are proportionately similar by their level of development measured in terms of the social amenities and level of development.

However, effort was made to identify the areas of differences or distinction amongst the people. Thus, a style of contrast in writing this brief ethnography was adopted.

9.2.2 Location, Land and Climate

The Sapele and Ethiope-East local government areas are two (2) of the existing twenty-five (25) local government areas in Delta state of Nigeria. They lie roughly between longitude 5° 00' and 6° 45' East and latitude 5° 00' and 6° 30' North. They both share common boundaries and are both accessible to each other by road or river transportation.

Climatically, the two local government areas share similar seasons like the large geographical entity called Nigeria. That is, the local governments areas are marked by two distinct seasons, the dry and rainy seasons.

The dry season occurs between the months of November and April, while the rainy season begins in the month of April and last till October. The average annual rainfall, in both areas is between 266.7cm and 190.5cm. Rainfall is heaviest in July, while high temperature ranges between 29°C and 44°C with an average put at 30°C in both areas[164]

The areas are low - lands and plains without ills or mountains. The vegetation ranges from mangrove swamps to minimal savannah. While Sapele local government area has a total landmass of 291.37 square miles, Ethiope-East local government has a land area of 742.5 square kilometres.

9.2.3. The People

The people of both local government areas share very strong similarities in social, economic, cultural and political characteristics. They speak corresponding languages, which has his common source from the 'Urhobo' language. However, while the people from Sapele local government area, speak a dialect called 'Okpe'. The people of Ethiope- East local government area could speak urhobo fluently and other borderline languages like 'Bini' and 'Itsekiri' due to border line proximity. In spite of these, there is a very high degree of mutual intelligibility amongst the people of both local government areas. This has been supported by a number of intelligent reports on claims to a common ancestor, identical traditional administrative systems as well as similar mode of traditional worships.[165]

Demographically, the population of Sapele local government area is put at 170,300. Though, the landmass is small in size, the local government area is one

---

[164] Government gazette on Local Governments Creation, Delta state information department, 1999.
[165] R. E. Bradbury and P.C. Llyord, 1957, Pp. 127-202.

of the most densely populated in the state. It is comprised of about six major communities namely, Sapele, Amukpe, Elume, Ogiede, Ugborhen and Ikeresan. However, the local government headquarter is located in the cosmopolitan town called Sapele.

On the other hand, Ethiope-East local government area, is made up of about 112, 000 people in about ten major communities, Ijenesa, Ajavwini, Ovadje, Mosogar, Jesse, etc. with headquarters at Jesse-town- A small town busy with a lot of commercial activities.

9.2.4. Polity

Both local government areas have a similar political structure, which is in line with the constitution of the Federal Republic of Nigeria. However, alongside with the governmental structure exist the monarchical system of traditional governance. They are recognized kings that head the traditional structure of leadership in the various communities. They perform both political and religious functions. While at the same time, they are regarded as the custodian of the people's culture. They are subject to the constitutional leaders or executives of their local governments referred to as Chairmen.

While in Sapele local government area, the king is referred to as 'Orodje'. In Ethiope-East local government, they are referred to as 'Ovie'. In both cases, they perform similar duties.[166]

In practical terms, the people of both local governments areas, owe their unalloyed allegiance first to their traditional rulers. The traditional institution commands more respect when compared to the official governmental structures. Most decisions are taken by governmental officials, in concerts with contributions of ideas from the traditional council.

The 'Orodje' and 'Ovies' administer their traditional territories with the support of their chiefs, who are referred to as 'Olorogun'. They also, have the traditional prime - minister, who is next in the hierarchy to the King. He is referred to traditionally as the 'Iyasere.' The town crier of the information officer is referred to as the 'Otota'. The other chiefs (Olorogun), also, play prominent roles in the Orodje and Ovie cabinet as requested from time to time.

On sensitive traditional and cultural matters the traditional institutions play very significant roles in these ethnic groups.

---

[166] Kingsley U. Omoyibo 1995, Unpublished M.Sc. thesis, Pp. 34-35

9.2.4.1. Traditional Administrative Structure of Sapele and Ethiope-East Local Government Areas of Delta State, Nigeria

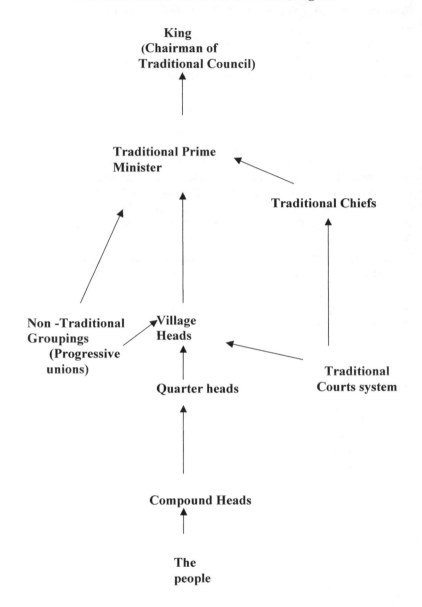

9.2.5. Economy

Both local government areas are subsistence economies. The areas are blessed with fertile land that can sustain farming throughout the year. The people engage in the cultivation of both subsistence and cash crops like, cassava, pepper, maize, plantain, oil palm, rubber, raffia palm, timber etc. The area also, has an extensive deposit of mineral resources like, crude oil (black gold) product.

Specifically, Sapele local government area is known for its cosmopolitan nature and importance for the existence of a Sea Port that is, important, for the trade in timber related products. This business is heavily influenced by the presence of the African Timber and Plywood (ATP) established by the Miller brothers in Sapele in 1935. The local government also, serves as a base for the Nigerian Navy.

Ethiope-East local government on its own is rich in mineral and forestry resources. The name Ethiope is derived from the river Ethiope that separate the local government area from Sapele. This river is noted for high level, commercial activities like fishing, and transportation of lumbering products, as well as for salt production. The people also, engage in high scale production of rubber products.

Although, there are existence of modern industrial and commercial enterprises in these areas, the people are also, often readily associated with agrarian activities like agriculture as their major occupation and reliable means of sustenance. While the women are more involved in agricultural cultivation, the men are mostly hunters for games and timber lumbering.

9.2.6. Social Organization

The existing communities in both local governments areas are patriarchal in nature. Emphasis is more on the extended family system that is rooted in the kinship units of society. As pointed out elaborately in the preceding work on social organizational structure of the many ethnic groups in Nigeria, many women are often made to play subordinate roles in these areas except for some very few that must have gone through certain requirements. They are considered inferior to men in line with what is said to be the long established customs of the people. This is evident from the fact that women must not sit at the same place and be talking at the same time with their husband, in the presence of family members or in-laws of the man except she was instructed to speak. This practice is very common among the Urhobo, Okpe and Isoko ethnic groups in the Delta areas of Nigeria.

In religious practices the people are divided along the three dominant religions namely, Christianity, Islam, and traditional beliefs. The traditional worship is presided over by the chief priest in concert with the traditional ruler (king).

Thus, the above form the veritable basis for organized social order in the various existing communities in both local government areas of research study.

9.2.7. Women and Sexuality amongst Urhobo and Okpe Ethnic Groups

Traditionally, women played the second fiddle role in both ethnic groups dominated by men. They took care of the home and children and had no equal opportunity like their male counterpart to be educated. Their role simply reduced to reproductive and procreation activities. They were more or less reproduction machines.

Women also were engaged in petty domestic activities like weaving, farming, fishing and trading. They were not allowed far away from home for fear of being seduced by other men or non-relatives. They only had close contacts with male family members like, brothers, father, or other male relations.

Marriage marked a transfer of allegiance from father to husband. Marriage was by patrilocal arrangement since the ethnic groups practiced a patrilineal system of social organization. Girls stayed at home most times until they were married except to accompany parents to perform some domestic household shores. Though, they were allowed minimal visits to female visitors, and to attend certain festivals for a brief period of time. Girls were not educated at this time except to learn some of the minimal form of education at home. Women had no political rights of any kind and were controlled by men at nearly every stage of their lives. Since men spent most of the time outside the house, home life, was dominated by the women from the Urhobo, Okpe and Isoko ethnic groups. She supervised the daily running of the household, took charge of raising the children, and does the cooking for the entire household as well as engaged in other task like weaving, sewing and other petty talent activities. Sometimes, she was effectively assisted by, her children or other relatives living with them.

As the female child grows, she was socialized about her sex and the attitudes, and behaviour that accompany her role and place in the society. The emphasis of the socialization was to equip her with the role she was going to play as a woman in the future different from those of men.

However, today, with enlightenment and awareness arising from modernization, women in these ethnic groups are now allowed access to education and career in the society. Many families are now interested in the training of female children. Though, this has somewhat improved the awareness and elevated the status of women, it did not however, changed the role of women in terms of their domestic and reproductive responsibilities and their subordinate status in these communities. With this educational opportunity opened to women, most of them have been able to perform equal or better than men, and this has created some psychological fears and role conflict between men and women at both the domestic and societal fronts in these ethnic societies. In spite, of these changes, women in the Urhobo and Okpe ethnic groups especially, remain a significant factor in the stability of the family. She provides love, sex and emotion to her husband and at the same time performs very cordial biological and social role in the maintenance of the children.

Amongst these ethnic groups, female circumcision is believed to enhance and improves marriage prospect. In fact, circumcision is considered to make the girl child eligible for marriage. More so, polygamy is a social norm that benefits the man to the detriment of the woman in these ethnic groups. While men are allowed the practice, it is a taboo for the woman to engage in polyandry.

At the communication front, women are subordinate to men. They are more of listeners to speakers at home. The men issued the authority and the women obeyed. The man is dominant and the woman is subservient in this respect. The woman however, plays the role of counselling and relieving stress at home during tensed and sensitive family issues. Though, today, men help in the care of children like the women, it is worthy to mention that at the young phase of the child development, mother relationship to the child is of high importance. In all, women still play subordinate roles in the Urhobo, Okpe, and Isoko ethnic groups.

10.0. Chapter ten
10.1. Presentation and Analysis of Data
This chapter deals with the presentation and analysis of data. The analysis is done to focus my research to meet the demand of the stated aims and objectives, hypotheses and the general assumptions on abortion, female circumcision, adolescent females reproductive health and other essential components of reproductive health systems, respectively in Nigeria. The analysis is descriptive with some simple quantitative remarks to illuminate it.

Table 10.1. **Data collection techniques and number of respondents / participants in each category**

Data Collection Techniques	Number of Respondents	Sex Distribution	
		Male	Female
Focus Group Discussion	27	10	17
Personal Interviews	15	7	8
Case Studies	2	-	2
Grand Total	**44**	**17**	**27**

Source: fieldwork, 2000 and 2001
The above table shows the distribution of respondents / participants in the multiple technique adopted for data collection. The break down reveal that the sample of distribution of participants in the categories adopted had more females than males. This was because the distribution was skewed to reflect the group whose opinion and involvement in matters of reproductive health - abortion and female circumcision are relevant to the aims and objectives of the study. The male opinion on the issues is to give the findings of this research a holistic and scientific explanation of the phenomena under study.

Table 10.1 a: Age categories of respondents / participants

Age categories (years)	Number of Respondents/ Participants	Sex Distribution	
		Male	Female
15 - 19	17	5	12
20 - 24	4	2	2
25 - 29	2	-	2
30 - 34	2	-	2
35 +	19	10	9
Grand Total	**44**	**17**	**27**

Source: Fieldwork, 2000 and 2001

The table above reveal the sharp classification or dichotomy between the ages of the adolescents who are the target especially the females and the older age categories. This helped to establish a reliable analysis of the differing views between both generations on the issues under study. Using the World Health Organization (WHO) definition of adolescents, youths and the aged, it is obvious from the above table that those between 15 and 24 years (classified as youths) are more in number when compared to the aged category (i.e. 35+.) This is a reflection of the purpose of this research that targets the adolescent opinion in particular.

Table 10.1 b: Ethnic composition of respondents / participants

Ethnic Composition	Number of Respondents/ Participants	Sex Distribution	
		Male	Female
Urhobo / Okpe	30	13	17
Agbor	3	1	2
Itsekiri	6	1	5
Bini	1	-	1
Isoko	1	1	-
Yoruba	1	1	-
Hausa	2	-	2
Grand Total	**44**	**17**	**27**

Source: fieldwork 2000 and 2001

The table above show the distribution of respondents / participants according to their ethnic group. Furthermore, it revealed the existence of the multi-ethnic nature of the research area under study. This ethnic composition helped in understanding the various ethnic groups cultural conceptions of the issues of abortion, female circumcision and other reproductive health issue. It also helped to establish areas of similarities and differences in their conception of the research issues.

Table 10.1 c: Religious composition of Respondents / Participants

Religious composition	Number of Respondents/ Participants	Sex Distribution	
		Male	Female
Christians	38	14	24
Muslims	2	-	2
Traditional Worshippers	4	3	1
Grand Total	**44**	**17**	**27**

Source: fieldwork 2000 and 2001

It is shown in the above table that there are more Christians than other forms of religious practitioners. This is explained in the context of the area of the research that is in the Southern part of Nigeria with a predominant Christian population. Religion in this context explains its influence in conditioning the cultural philosophies and behaviour of the people. It should be noted however, that most of the Christians and Islamic followers are equally strong adherents of traditional religious practices. Hence, the few numbers recorded in the category of traditional worshippers were those who openly expressed their opinion in that respect. They could be more in the context in which I have explained above.

Table 10.1 d: Level of Educational attainment of the respondents / participants

Educational Qualification	Number of Respondents/ Participants	Sex Distribution	
		Male	Female
Not Educated	5	3	2
Elementary School	2	1	1
Secondary / College, (JSS, SSS)	19	6	13
Secondary (incomplete)	2	1	1
Diploma, NCE, other higher certificate.	7	1	6
University and above	9	5	4
Grand Total	**44**	**17**	**27**

Source: fieldwork 2000 and 2001

The table shows clearly that the target population (adolescents) were either still in schools or graduated from colleges already (see Appendix I). However, there were a few who could not complete their colleges as shown for reasons ranging from inability to finance their education or victim of unwanted pregnancy. The participant level of education had a tremendous impact on their conceptualisation of the theme of the research.

10.2. Conception of respondents on Sex
10.2.1. Adolescent Views
Adolescents hold that sex before marriage or pre-marital sex is bad. They point to the issue of the negative consequences of it. They listed some of these consequences as the issue of social responsibility, unwanted pregnancy, contraction of sexually transmitted diseases and the effect on their education. This is encapsulated on the extract of a discussion below:

(I):	...what is your conception of sex?
(K):	...when a male and female come together to engage in sexual intercourse...it is a very deep relationship...it should be established only after marriage, doing it before marriage is very bad...the problem with doing it before marriage are more likely unwanted pregnancy....
(C):	(cut in rudely)...as for me sex before marriage is illegitimate sex...apart from unwanted pregnancy mentioned by (K), most other girls have died from the perpetuation of abortion, some others abandoned school and became useless...sex is only meant for married couples...
(E):	Sex is only bad when you are not up to the stage...

Though the general consensus was that sex before marriage has serious consequences. But the consensus opinion amongst adolescents is that sex is not bad when and if both parties involved are matured enough to handle the responsibilities that emanates from the consequences. They view sex as another way of cementing a relationship. This point is emphasised more by male adolescents as in the excerpt below:

| (M) | ...sex is a confirmation of an established affection between the boy and the girl. It also helps to cool down mental stress... |
| (I) | ...I think sex before marriage has advantages. It prepares the boy and the girl for the future ...both acquire experiences that make future marriages last longer. Sex and satisfaction goes hand in hand. It guaranties marital stability in the future. |

The above suggest that sex for the average adolescent male plays both biological and social functions.[167] The issue of satisfying sexual instincts and helping to solidify social relationships and avoid a future break in marital relationship in the future. This help to stabilize society from incessant divorces. In this context, there is a social acceptance of pre-marital sex amongst adolescent.

Some of the common terms used for sex by adolescent include, 'banging', 'poking', 'fucking', 'screwing', 'yanshing', 'filing' etc. The adolescent males use common terms to classify different forms of sexual partners like, girl friends, babies, wife, and bed- mate. While terms like boy friends, lover, sugar daddies, fuck mates are common terms used by adolescent females.

---

[167] Carla Makhlouf Obermeyer 1994, Pp. 74-75.

Adolescent female suggested age ranges of 18 to 20 years, and 20 to 22 years for females and males respectively before starting to have sex. They theorized their point on biological facts conditioned by improvement in social circumstances that makes the female develop faster than their male counterparts. The adolescent males contended this point by suggesting that the ages of between 18 to 20 years and 20 to 22 years for male and female respectively. When asked why? The following extracts of the discussion held,

(I):   what are your reasons for the above classification....

(OV):   because boys are more experienced and matured on issues of sex than girls no matter if they were younger. I cannot explain further but *that is just the way it is*...

(K):   I think for girls it should be between 20 and 22 years ... *it is just adequate to my mind*...

The above responses reveal the gender nature of the males and a reflection of sex preference during the process of socialization in the society that culturally make them to believe that they are superior to the female on issues that pertains to sex. The use of the terms, 'I cannot explain further', 'that is just the way it is', 'it is just adequate to my mind' are reflections of languages of cultural superiority imposed by many Urhobo, Okpe, Isoko, Agbor and Bini cultures on men to the disadvantage of the female child. These reinforces old prejudices about male superiority in the society[168]

Though there is a consensus position amongst adolescent males and females on the illegality or non- approval of sex before marriage. On critical evaluation, there is a high priority placed by respondents on the issue of sex before marriage. This implies a level of expectation or a degree of acceptance of pre-marital sex. This position was further amplified when a question was posed to all adolescent on; who amongst them have had sex? The males reacted in the positive and some even claimed to have had it very regularly. But when the same question was posed to the females, their initial response was a 'dead silence' and murmurings. On a reframed question as to, who amongst them was still a virgin? None accepted to have been a virgin at that point in time. Their attitude to such question maybe because the researcher is a male or as a result of the cultural backgrounds, which makes women shy and uncomfortable discussing sexual habits in the presence of males other than their boy friends, husbands, or close confidants like peer groups and friends.[169] In fact, all the adolescent females in the discussion group, including those with very strong Christian beliefs identified during the group discussion, and case study sessions acknowledged not been virgins.

In effect, adolescents may be opposed openly to pre-marital sexual activities. But the suggested ideal ages at first sexual experiences, and their response to the

---

[168] Reuben Abati, 'Two widows, Lam and Akume.' Guardian Newspaper online, Friday March 15, 2002, www.ngrguardiannews.com accessed on March 15, 2002.
[169] U. Linke 1986, Pp. 203.

virginity question is consistent with the existing reality. This conflicting view of adolescents between 'theory' and 'practice' may partly explain the hesitation to publicly support adolescent reproductive health programmes in Nigeria, leaving a fragile foundation on which to build such initiative.[170]

10.2.2. Adult Views

Sex is done for two purposes. First it is seen as a pre-requirement for reproduction- that is, to reproduce or to produce children. Second, sex is done for pleasure. Adults view sex as a veritable determinant or proof of fertility. Among the Urhobo, Okpe, Bini, Itsekiri, Agbor and Isoko cultures the ability to have a child, and a significant proof of fertility is commenced first through sexual intercourse. This is otherwise, known as sex.

Adults view sex as a sacred act. To them it is a taboo to have sex before marriage. Thus sex is seen as an act that is socially regulated. Though there are exceptional cases where sex before marriage are allowed, such situations occasionally occurs.

Adults view sexual taboos as follows,

- to pronounce the name of sex organs
- to expose the sex organ unnecessarily
- taboo for a woman to say to a man 'come and sex me'
- taboo to be nursing a baby and having sex
- taboo to have sex during menstruation
- taboo to be pregnant without marriage
- taboo to have sex with certain degree of relations (rule of incest and exogamy) etc

Adults emphasised on the indiscriminate form of pre-marital sex amongst today's adolescents particularly the females. They identified a number of factors that accounts for the indiscriminate pre- marital sex in the society. Some of the factors listed include, poverty, parental laxity in the discipline of their children, peer group influences, weakened societal values, influence of western civilization, un-circumcision of females etc. This is summed up in an excerpt of a discussion with adults:

> (I): ...How do you perceive adolescents and sex ...
>
> (ME): In my view, nowadays boys and girls are so loosed In this sex of a thing. In the olden days you hardly see an unmarried girl holding hands or moving freely with boys...today they feel that it is only when you engage in sex that you could be referred to as civilized---
>
> (JE): ... in the olden days if an unmarried boy and girl were caught in sex acts they were seriously beaten publicly. These cherished values are now dead because of what is called *civilization*. In fact, young girls are now engaged in sex anyhow because of money- for may be #100.00 a small girl

---

[170] NCPD and JHU/PCS, KNIECSS, 1994

> would open her legs and get sexed badly.../ this is what is responsible for various sexually transmitted diseases ...in those days before engaging in sexual relationship couples must be married...

(AO): The backgrounds of children affect their upbringing...so you find out that since most of today Children particularly, the girls are not well brought up, they misbehave. So when somebody just call them on the streets for a meagre sum of money they fall victim of sex prey...it is very sad...

The above expressions exposes the myth tied around the issue of sex in traditional and cultural societies. Adults still believe that issue of the virginity of the female used to be a very priced value among the Urhobo, Itsekiri and Okpe customs. However, today 'female virginity' is not any more, much of traditional moral factor, but fundamental Christian moral issue. Researches had shown that earlier lack of scientific knowledge and cultural taboos on sex talk impeded people from freely talking about sex related issues particularly as it affected the female body in traditional societies.[171] Adult respondents decried the fading away of this otherwise one time cherished value as enthused by Chief J in the excerpt below:

(CJ): in the time of old, girls go to marriages with their virginity and honour; it was a very priced value. But regrettably, this is not any more because of promiscuity. It is not wrong to say that we are more immoral now than before...because some of us the parents even accommodates bastard children from illicit relationships...

Thus adults engaged themselves in trans-generational comparison of traditional versus modernity. They were nostalgic of the good old days. It was their opinion that 'modernization and westernisation' influence like education, modern economy, television, obscene film shows with wild acts such as rapes and violent crimes has contributed a lot to what they termed the 'sexual immorality' of today's adolescents.[172]

Adults were however of the consensus view that sex can only be recommended when the individuals were legally married. To them it did not matter whether adolescents were younger than 18 years or not. In fact, Madam (O) put it this way:

(MO): when a girl is about 15 years old, men can seek her hand in marriage and the moment she is married whether she is younger or older the issue of sex could be engaged in...they could be regarded as responsible for whatever actions of theirs pertaining to sex and other family responsibilities. I was personally given out in marriage at the age of 14 and today I am 60 years old...

---

[171] Irvine 1999, Pp. 162.
[172] Ogor Alubo 2000, Pp. 4-6.

Adults also identified the socio-economic condition of the country as a critical reason affecting most young men not to be able to engage in early marriages and consequently make them to seek pre-marital sex as a very great relief and the only alternative to satisfy their 'biological and social' desires out of wedlock. This same socio-economic condition has been used to explain parental laxity in terms of the neglect of discipline and proper upbringing of children to the pursuance of means of survival because of the harsh economic times. Also, many adolescent females engage in indiscriminate sex to earn incomes in order to cater for themselves and families due to the harsh socio-economic conditions, and neglecting the detriment of the dire health dangers that they may be exposed to. Studies have shown in this respect, that adolescent sexuality cannot be understood in isolation of the socio-economic, political and religious framework of the society.[173]

Adults believe that despite the degeneration of moral values and the demystification of sex by contemporary improvement in scientific knowledge and technological developments, some aspects of traditional cherished values and morals should be re-evaluated to maintain sanity in the system. They unanimously hold that young people should be taught about some aspect of sex educations and that the females should be specifically targeted. More so, they suggest that issues to be discussed must be 'selective' and not what would expose adolescents to more sexual immorality. They highlighted areas where emphasis should be focused on as, unwanted pregnancies, sexually transmitted diseases, HIV/AIDS infections, illegal abortion and not the encouragement of the use of contraceptives by adolescents.

10.2.3. Expert Views

They see sex as a normal human process that precedes reproduction. Medically, they are of the view that adolescents are much more sexually active at that stage of development. Adolescents to them engage in sex acts without adequate precautions like protecting themselves against socio-medical vices like unwanted pregnancy, abortions, infectious sexual diseases and the contraction of the ultimate known sexual disease the HIV/AIDS virus. The study of Okonofua, et al. (1999) on sexually transmitted diseases among Nigerian adolescents confirms the opinion of experts.[174]

The experts observed from their practical experience the rampancy of sex amongst contemporary Nigerian adolescents when compared to about a decade ago. Though they condemn in strict terms pre-marital sex, but hold that it would be very difficult to control. Experts recommended the ages between 18 and 20 years for adolescent maturity before engaging in sexual activities. They were of the opinion that at this age adolescents especially the females were physically, psychologically, physiologically and biologically matured and strong to embark

---

[173] Ogor Alubo 2000, Pp.6
[174] Friday E. Okonofua, et al. 1999, Pp. 184-186.

on reproductive activities without much danger. Experts recommended 20 years and above for males. For them it is a biological fact that, women develop faster and rapidly than their male counterparts.

The experts emphasized on the management of indiscriminate sex amongst adolescents, through education and access to the use of contraceptive. Since they should be no pretence that adolescents do engage in experimentation of sex at this age. This is encapsulated in the interview of one of them below:

> (I): when do you think it is most appropriate for adolescents to have sex...
>
> (Bea): customarily, it would have been better for pre-marital sex to be discouraged...but this is going to be very difficult at the adolescent stage and this era of modernity. So the very best thing to do is to manage the problem by way of enlightening these adolescents to be aware of certain dangers ...Parents should have a lot to do in this respect.

Thus experts de-emphasize cultural and traditional myths that are used to becloud sex issues and acknowledge the need for the use of enlightenment and education to increase the awareness of adolescents about the inherent dangers that emerges from a number of reproductive health problems. This is consistent with earlier studies by Alubo Ogor on adolescent reproductive health in Nigeria.[175] The unorthodox health experts held similar views like those of the adolescents in this perspective.

10.3. Conception of Respondents on Abortion, Contraception and its Consequences
10.3.1. Adolescent Views

Adolescents recognized unwanted pregnancy as a very common phenomenon amongst them, and that most of the victims are unmarried adolescent females. Though just two out of the twelve adolescent females accepted to have had personal experiences with the circumstances of unwanted pregnancy; the other ten agreed to have had indirect experiences with the circumstances as shown in the excerpt of the discussion below:

> (I):   Have you ever been pregnant?
>
> (EA): I have never been pregnant, but I know most of my friends who are very young who had. But they aborted the thing...
>
> (OK): eh! eh! I know of many friends who had been pregnant but they terminated them locally in one traditional clinic around Okpe road, here in Sapele. But I will not mention the place, and some others did theirs at a popular private clinic here in town...

---

[175] Ogor Alubo 2000, Pp. 2.

Reasons are bound why adolescents do not accept to have had personal experiences and perform the act in secret. Some of these include, the fear of prosecution and the social stigma that the information relating to abortion carries by both the client and provider in the society.[176]

Adolescents are not educated on the legal provisions or implications that prohibits the procurement of abortion. Much of what they know about illegal abortion has to do with information from unclear sources like hear-say, fellow school mates, peer groups, friends[177] and epileptic by-lines information of abortion cases in newspapers, and much more from cultural, traditional and religious theologies and teachings, which claim that deliberate spilling of blood like the issue of aborting unwanted pregnancy is murder and sin against God and man. This particular mode of teaching propel adolescents females in Benin, Sapele and Jesse town to terminate unwanted pregnancy clandestinely and obtain such services from untrained professionals in environments failing to meet basic minimal medical standards. Most of such abortions are considered unsafe.[178]

In an excerpt of discussions with adolescent males, three out of five of them accepted to have taken their pregnant girl friends at one or more times to trado-medical homes or quacks (chemist operators) to procure abortion for the fear of been apprehended by law enforcement agents in recognized public health and even private health institutions. The excerpt below expresses the point clearly,

(I):   Has any of you here had a girl friend that was Pregnant…?

(D, R, K): # yes #...

(I):   what happened to it?

(D, R, K): #aborted of course #

(A):   (cut in), but for me I decided that my girl friend should have it, because I know that God shall provide…

(I):   how did you people abort that of your girl friends- D, R, K?

(ED):   I have done at least two of such abortion for my girl friend. I did it in a herbal home where she was given some mixture of herbs to insert into her private part to allow the child to dissolve…

(UR):   My girl friend was given a mixture of local gin and Codeine tablets. It was recommended by a friend as a very effective means of expelling pregnancy…at

---

[176] Thapa Shyam and Padhye M. Saraswati 2001, Pp. 146.

[177] International Planned Parenthood Federation (IPPF) / United Nations Population Fund (UNFPA); Generation 97-What young people say about sex and reproductive health, 1997

[178] Unsafe abortion is defined by the WHO as a procedure for terminating an unwanted pregnancy either by persons lacking the necessary skills or in an environment lacking the minimal medical standards or both. (WHO: The Prevention and Management of Unsafe Abortion; Report of a Technical Working Group, WHO/MSM/92.5, 1992.)

other times, I bought menstrogen injection liquid mixed with hot gin for my girlfriend to drink…On one occasion she bled seriously, at other times it came just very easy and cool…

(K): I wanted to do it at a private clinic for my girl friend but the cost was to expensive for me to bear so I had to adopt the local approach. This I did after using a combination of failed drugs like Prostinol, and menstrogen I bought at the chemist…

The excerpt of the above discussion show, that most adolescents have engaged in perpetuating abortions for their girl friends more than once and they seek ideas of termination of unwanted pregnancy from their contemporaries or from other informal sources. More so, adolescent intention to go to public hospitals and recognized health centres to seek such services are impaired by their apprehension for the law.[179] While those with enough courage complain of costly charges of the doctors in private clinics who offer such services. Evidence are bound that even most abortion service providers are not adequately trained and equipped and thus lack in the skill of providing quality services. This account for the dangerous, and in most cases fatal procedures adopted in conducting abortion issues. This is also evident in the study of Otoide, et al. (2001) on why adolescent seek abortion rather than contraception.[180]

Though two out of the twelve adolescent females agreed to have had a personal experience with unwanted pregnancy and the issue of abortion, the other ten informed that they had at one or more times missed their monthly periods and influenced its flow by taking self medicated drugs, consulted with quacks, chemist attendants, discussed with friends, and sometimes with traditional herbalists to recommend a combination of herbal mixtures. While some of these processes proved effective for seven of the adolescent females, the others ended up in the hospitals with related illnesses arising from complications, which was reported as cases of fever illnesses at hospitals. This again emphasizes the secrecy that beclouds issues of abortion due to the restrictive law in place.

Discussion amongst adolescent revealed, general opposition to abortion in the open, but in practical reality the opposite prevail. When asked why most of them induce periods or engage in aborting? The adolescent males gave reasons such as, 'I am too young to be a father', I needed to further my career', 'I do not think I would want to marry that girl in future and 'I do not want to start a polygamous family', I do not want my parents to stop fending for me because of my additional responsibilities' etc. While adolescent females gave reasons for aborting pregnancy as, 'the baby's father refusing responsibility', 'inability to cater for the child alone', pregnancy resulting from rape', 'rejection of them by their parents and the withdrawal of all parental care and responsibility' etc.

---

[179] Tony B. E. Ogiamen 1991, Pp. 125-126.
[180] Valentine Otoide 2001, Pp. 80.

Adolescent knowledge of contraceptive usage to prevent pregnancy is limited. Although most of them (especially males) are aware of the use of condoms for the prevention of unwanted pregnancy and the contraction of sexually transmitted diseases, but unfortunately do not find it convenient to use it during sex acts. This is contrary to earlier research the findings.[181] Only one out of the five adolescent males accepted a regular usage of the condom during sex. The others claim they trust their girl friends, and still others believe that it does not make them to enjoy sex. It was their opinion that when it is natural, it is better. The excerpt from (AO) and
(KO) put it succinctly as thus:

(AO): I do not take any pills or use any form of protective stuff like condom / I trust my babe...I do not even know how to wear the condom although I see it regularly. Truly I do not like it...

(KO): Rather than use the condom for love - making, I take a combination of drugs like tetracycline, ampiclux capsules...

(I): but assuming your girl friend insists you wear a condom...?

(UR): (cut in rudely)...*she cannot say that.* I will ask her to go away and I will go to my other girl friends...

(KO): I have made my girl friend to understand that, that is the only way I enjoy sex with her, and she on her own understands. So there is no problem...

On protective sex, ten out of the twelve adolescent females said they rely on counting 'safe periods' and the 'withdrawal system' as some of the effective mechanisms or devices for preventing unwanted pregnancy. The common reason given by them was that their boy friends preferred to have sex with them the natural way in order for them (males) to enjoy it. This process of Natural Family Planning (NFP), which sometimes could prove unreliable because most of them do not count it right or get confused in the process of counting, has been identified in a previous study of adolescent reproductive health in Kenya (NCPD/JHU/PCS, 1994). This was identified, when they were asked to specify when their safe period was. Studies have also shown the inefficacy of the withdrawal system. The excerpts below reveal some of the responses,

(I): why don't you insist on condom from your boy...?

(EE): (Laugh Long!!!)- He does not like it...moreover, I cannot say no because I know he has other girl friends and my saying no will make him leave me. It is very difficult to get a boy friend easily nowadays...so I prevent myself by counting periods

---

[181] Valentine Otoide 2001, Pp. 79.

	or taking some form of combination of drugs with alcohol...
(T):	I do it myself by counting my menstrual period. So far, it has helped me a lot. My boyfriend does not cooperate.
(I):	why don't you educate your boy friends...?
(T):	they never understand and you know a girl is weak to say no because it may cause a lot of harm to the relationship...
(R):	'whenever my boy friend is coming during sex act, he withdraws it immediately so that the sperm does not get inside me...that is how we do it...but if pregnancy result by error, he is the first person that will say that it should be aborted totally...though, it has never happened, but he said that is what will be done if it ever happens...'

The above expressed views show male control of sexual relationship. The females are at the mercy of their male counterparts who dictate the entire pace of sexual behaviour and relationship.[182] However, females are more tolerant of the resultant consequences of unprotected sex- pregnancy and abortion, and contraction of sex diseases than their male counterparts. The male consideration of 'self' and immediate pleasure override the sense of rational judgement when the consequences result. For instance, four out of the five adolescent males said they would accept abortion outright if their girl friend were pregnant at any point in time. Only one agrees to accept the baby, be delivered. Seven adolescent females would prefer to have the baby if the boyfriend accepts responsibility, and in most cases the boy never does. This is contrary to the findings of JHU/PCS studies carried out among Kenya adolescents in 1994.

Religious inclinations of adolescent significantly influence their ideas about unwanted pregnancy and the procurement of abortion as well as the use of contraceptives. Ten out of seventeen adolescents condemned unwanted pregnancy, abortion and the use of contraceptives for the prevention of abortion, from a strict religious standpoint. It was their views that it is a sin and highly immoral in the sight of God. This view is similar to that held by pro- life activists that it is a sin to commit abortion in whatever form and for whatever reasons.[183] However, their beliefs are contradictory when matched with the reality and practice amongst them.

Adolescents acknowledged complications and deaths resulting from abortions procured to get rid of unwanted pregnancy by their very close relations, friends, neighbours, school- mates etc. Many of them accepted (14 of them) that young people should be allowed unlimited access to the procurement of contraceptives to prevent unwanted pregnancy and abortion.

---

[182] Carla Makhlouf Obermeyer 1994, Pp.54
[183] Randy Alcorn 1992, Pp. 1 and Frederica Mathews-Green 1994, Pp. 1-4.

10.3.2. Adult views on Abortion, Contraception its Consequences

Adult conceive that abortion when not induced or miscarriage is a sure proof of fertility and also a sign of other unhealthy conditions in woman or both. Abortion or miscarriage committed on purpose is regarded as killing and a cultural crime. In effect any form of induced abortion done for any reason by any individual is abomination and has a devastating spiritual consequences. Such culprits are accused of having poured human blood on earth and the earth must be purified. This is also evident in the findings of Micheal Angulu Onwuejeogwu study of women's reproductive health among the Igbo people of South-East Central Nigeria.[184]

Adult reason that modernization and the introduction of certain form of technological aids like the Television, Radio and even western education has facilitated the weakening of traditional value and morality. For instance, sex that used to be mystified is now an open adoration. The increase in the rate of unwanted pregnancy, abortions, as well as sexually transmitted diseases by adolescent has been attributed to these modern trends.

Further more, they hold that adolescents abuse sex without taking adequate precautions. To them, this creates unnecessary burden on society in the form of increase in social vices- like prostitution, robbery and other dangerous unclassifiable crimes. Instead of abortion, adult conceive an effective social welfare system to be put in place to cater for those with unwanted pregnancies. Their position is encapsulated in the views expressed by Madam Onem,

> (MO): to kill is a sin and abortion is killing. It is better for girls who are pregnant to have the baby and their parents to take responsibility or else the social welfare unit should take care of such responsibilities...it would make parents to sit up and exercise discipline over their children instead of pursuing wealth...it will teach the girl the language of responsibility when she sees the liability she has caused ...it is better for her to avoid multiple suicide by committing abortion...

Adult believe that the position above has three basic advantages. First, it would create the willingness for parents to exercise control over their children; second, it will prevent deaths that result from the procurement of illegal abortion; and third, it will allow the victim to have the baby and help teach the adolescent involved the language of responsibility. In all of these, one of the dissenting adult, views the female as the worst victim. This adult observed that such a situation would place the male in an advantaged position to keep wrecking havoc on innocent female victims. This view is express by Mr. W, in the excerpt below,

> (W): both the boy and the girl should be made to bear full responsibility and not the girl alone...the

---

[184] Michael A. Onwuejeogwu 2000, Pp. 33.

> boy should be taught a serious lesson of not creating liability for society. He should be given a serious job to do to earn income and cater for the responsibility he has created. By the time he combined job, school and the management of family, he would learn to be responsible…

The position of Mr. W draws attention to the gender division in addressing sex issues amongst male and female adolescents, that often made the girl child the victim at all times. However, adults acknowledge without pretence that adolescents are very sexually active at this stage of development and see it as a proper development for parents, teachers and society to educate them on the dangers of engaging into early parenthood. This is also reported in the studies of Nare, C. et al. (1997).[185] The excerpt from this discussant summed it up,

> (M): sex issues should be discussed with children when they attain puberty…my parents denied me of such and it did not help. I pardon them because they were illiterates. But today, times have changed. The earlier we make them to know about certain issues the better for us, and the society. We cannot prevent them from sex issues. They see it all around… let us save the situation…

Adult accept the above position with caution, that adolescents should only be taught when they are old enough. They claim this would help the grown up ones to discuss certain unusual body occurrence with their parents when it does arose. For instance Mr. Egbo illustrated this in his discussion,

> (E): …my daughter of 15 years saw her menses for the first time and shouted with scare that she was bleeding. We (mother) could have saved the situation if we told her earlier to expect such in the process of development of the child. These are little things that we hide that should be changed to prevent embarrassment. But abortion should not be encouraged…

Adults were sceptical about the introduction and distribution of contraceptives for preventives, like condoms and pills to adolescents as part of the educating and enlightenment process. They entertain the fear that it would expose them to much abuse and encourage a dangerous trend of sex escapade without limit, and that the essence is not to do that. They advocated that the best form of education of contemporary adolescent should be the emphasis on sex abstinence and the dangers of early sexual experience rather than introducing their access to the use of modern contraceptives.

10.3.3. Expert views on Abortion, Contraception and its Consequences

These views cover both the orthodox and unorthodox health expert practitioners. This researcher showed aspects where significant differences occurred.

---

[185] C. Nare, et al. 1997, Pp. 23.

The experts hold that reckless sex has become a high rate phenomenon among adolescents and that this accounts for the increase in unwanted pregnancy and illegal abortion among this sensitive category of individuals. They are of the view that they embark on sex without adequate precautions against known socio-medical vice which include the spread of dangerous sexual diseases like the HIV/AIDS. This is supported by findings from previous studies on adolescent reproductive health by Alubo, O. Okonofua, F.E. and Otoide, V. et al.[186]

Further more, orthodox expert practitioners hold that most adolescent females end up perpetuating dangerous abortions in abortion clinics because the act is illegal. The existence of the law banning abortion has encouraged patronage of quacks, nurses, traditional herbalist, and even established doctors not adequately skilled in the act of carrying out abortion.[187] The consequence has been the tremendous number of unrecorded deaths resulting from dangerously and criminally performed abortions.[188] It is the perspective of the orthodox health expert that adolescents be enlightened and encouraged to engage in protective sex and be allowed free accessibility to the use of contraceptives like condoms for males and pills for females. In an excerpt of interview with Dr. J, he reveal thus,

> (Dr. J.): this is because, if you recommend absolute
> abstinence from sex according to culture and
> tradition, you and I know that it won't work. A
> more realistic proposal is to advise and encourage
> contraceptive usage, and condom is the
> commonest…

Orthodox health experts blamed government for the restriction of adolescents to the procurement of contraceptive. They clarified the point that contraceptives help in preventing abortion, and that it would be better to prevent abortion rather than curing complications arising there from. They blame fanatical religious position of Christianity, Islam and traditional worshippers as major obstacles to the proposal for legislation on the procurement of legal abortion. In their view this is a dangerous trend for a country where about one-quarter of her population are in this sensitive brackets of adolescents.[189]

They hold a common position with their unorthodox health expert counterparts that the wide spread socio-economic hardship is a strong factor propelling indiscriminate sex among adolescent females for the purpose of survival. More so, this extends to the seeking for cheap process of procuring abortion in the case of eventual occurrence of unwanted pregnancy. This makes them to end up with quacks and the resultant dangers.

---

[186] Ogor Alubo 2000, Pp.2-4, / Friday E. Okonofua 1999, Pp. 185, / Valentine Otoide, et al. 2001, Pp. 77-81.
[187] Thapa Shyam and Padhye M. Saraswati, 2001, Pp. 144
[188] IFPP 2001, Pp. 147.
[189] Ogor Alubo 2000, Pp. 6-7.

There is an altercation between orthodox and unorthodox health expert practitioners views on the providers of such dangerous abortions. There is the passing of blames on each other in terms of the greatest accomplices in the act. Orthodox health expert practitioners blame many complicated abortions to the act performed by unorthodox health expert. While unorthodox health practitioners blamed the orthodox health providers for the same offence. This bulk passing by both expert health providers denying their involvement in or practice of illegal abortion could be explained in the context of the law that restricts abortion practice in Nigeria. This is consistent with earlier findings.[190] More so, the unorthodox health practitioners emphasized their opposition to any form of legislation meant to legalize or liberalise abortion as 'it is against tradition, culture and religion of the Urhobo, Okpe, Itsekiri and Bini speaking tribes to take a life that one cannot create.' They are of the view that sex should be sacred until parties where legitimately married. In spite, of these views, unorthodox practitioners hold that there are traditional contraceptive methods to prevent unwanted pregnancy. However, they cautioned and claim to administer such to female who were legally married with the consent of their husbands; and adolescent females with the consent of their parents especially, the father. It is noted in the above context, that fertility and reproductive health matters and decisions are not only dictated by the culture, but also by the social forces and power relationships in the family and the society at large. Thus men are favoured in this relationship to the detriment of women.[191] The excerpt from Chief Oko below explains the situation better,

> (CO): 'it is not easy for you to procure traditional contraceptives for the prevention of pregnancy. We only prepare it for married women with the consent of their husbands. While we prepare for young girls with the consent of their parents especially their father…I am a traditional man and so do not take culture for granted or else these children would abuse the process.'

The specialists hold the consensus view that abortion is very common among adolescent females, and that this results from laxity in parental control, widespread economic hardship, reckless and unprotected sex, waning of traditional values of morality due to modernization and technological influences, and the lack of awareness of adolescent on sex related issues. This is consistent with findings of earlier study on reproductive health of adolescent by Ogor Alubo.[192]

---

[190] Valentine Otoide et al. 2001, Pp. 80.
[191] Carla Makhlouf Obermeyer 1994, Pp. 59.
[192] Ogor Alubo 2000, Pp. 20-22.

10.4. Conception of Respondents on Legislative Policy on Abortion and Contraception

10.4.1. Adolescent Views

Adolescents are poorly equipped with the knowledge of the law on abortion and contraceptive usage. This makes them to rely on indirect sources of information on abortion and contraceptive usage. More so, due to the complete lack of awareness and the reliance on indirect sources of information, adolescent females resort to illegal processes for the procurement of abortion; and even when their lives is in danger from complicated, crude and dangerously perpetuated abortions they do not know how to go about it.[193] Consequently, most victims are damaged permanently for life or the unfortunate ones lose their lives in the process.

Despite the resulting complications from illegal abortion, opinions among adolescents were divided on the issue of the legalization or liberalization of abortion. About four out of seventeen adolescent respondents rejected completely any law to legalize abortion. Their views are expressed in the discussion below:

> (MA): ...I do not support at all any law on legalization of abortion. It is against Christianity...it is murder and it would encourage a number youths to engage in indiscriminate sex...it is a sin in the sight of God...
>
> (OG): ...it is a not biblical...I rebuke any such laws...
>
> (JT): as for me, abortion is likened to a hired assassin and Exodus chapter 20 verse 13 says, 'thou shall not kill'...
>
> (ES): the danger involve in such law is that, if care is not taken the girl and the child may lose their lives...

Religious and cultural beliefs are a strong influence on the views of adolescent females who oppose any such legislation on abortion. However, the contending adolescents who support legalization argued their point on the basis of reducing deaths of both mother and child perpetuated through illegal abortion and the need to control the number of quacks in the business of illegal abortion and help allow access of all female to proper medical care in the case of any such problem like unwanted pregnancy, and the need to procure qualitative abortion services at a very reduced cost by clients in the hands of expert practitioners. Some of the adolescent views are reflected underneath,

> (OK): legalizing abortion would help to reduce deaths that result from baby mothers and the patronage of quacks who mix all forms of combination of drugs for the girl to drink. It would also reduce the charges of doctors who perpetuate it because of the risk involved. All of this means better health---------
>
> (EL): I see it as a form of assistance to the whole girls in town because girls won't be ashamed anymore to walk to the doctor and do it...they can now get cheap access to

---

[193] F. Olowu 2001, Pp. 59-60

contraceptives to take care of themselves. It would reduce teenage deaths from unwanted pregnancy. I really support it...

(T.): I have seen girl friends of mine mixing local gin and tablets to rid off unwanted pregnancies because of the fear of going to an established clinic. All this would stop...even the patronage of traditional herbalist would stop...but government should impose some conditions before abortions should be procured so that the law is not abused...

(MI): it would create equal opportunity for all- both the rich and the poor girl to have access to the procurement of abortion and even contraceptive...

In fact, the issue of legalized abortion helping to sanitize society, and reducing the attitude of self medicated abortion drugs because of the fear of females going to public hospitals to request for abortion and the health of the mother was further emphasized in the above discussions. They also emphasized the need for the process to be controlled by stating conditions under which abortion should be allowed, so that it was not abused, and the need for creating equal accessibility to all females to procure abortion when they met with the required conditions.[194]

All adolescent males supported the idea of legalizing or liberalizing abortion. The major contentions came from the adolescent females themselves. Four out of the five adolescent males agreed to have perpetuated abortion for their girl friends through illegitimate means. They reported very unpleasant experiences in some of the instances.

The seventeen adolescents attested to have known female victims, who have been victims of illegally perpetuated abortions and some who died in the process. They claimed that victims were close relations, friends, neighbours, classmates, sister etc.

10.4.2. Adult views on Legislative Policy on Abortion and Contraceptives

Adults are aware of the laws on illegal abortion. They hold that the law is in concert with the traditional and cultural beliefs and practices of the people, and that deliberate termination of the foetus or 'induce miscarriage' of any form was treated as murder. It is the adult belief that abortion is traditionally, religiously and morally wrong. Thus they are in compromise with the Nigerian Criminal Law and Constitution on the banning of abortion. Adults blame the increase in the rate of deaths resulting from the abortion of unwanted pregnancy especially among adolescent females to the ineffective implementation of the law banning the practice. Studies on abortion in Nigeria have shown that the law banning its procurement has been ineffective, as the practice still continues clandestinely.[195] Two of the discussants summed it up in this form,

---

[194] Friday E. Okonofua et al. 1999, Pp. 189.
[195] Lukas Adetokumbo 1991, Pp. 14.

102

(W): ...those who are known to have collaborated to commit abortion (doctors and clients) in the past have not been arrested nor prosecuted. How then do you think the perpetrators of this criminal act especially adolescents would be deterred? /...The law is ineffective and weak...

(FO): ...as for me, I think that the government makes the laws and do not implement them ...how do you want the people to be serious?

These positions converges the views of the adults. They believe that legalizing or liberalizing abortion would increase the level of promiscuity among the youths.

Adults are resolute on their opposition to total legalization or liberalization of abortion. They contend that the issue is more than the proposed law, and that government should rather improve on the socio-economic status of women in particular, to enable them become self- reliant and independent to cope with survival needs instead of seeking unconventional approach to earning income like prostitution, or easy sex with the wide dimension of dire consequences.[196] Mrs. Imen stated it in this form:

"...Whether you liberalize the laws on abortion or not, if poverty as it affects the girl child is not eradicated in the country and my own community, we will still remain where we are...it is poverty that is the root of this whole thing call indiscriminate sex, prostitution, unwanted pregnancy, abortion and the contraction of diseases...

The emphasis by adults on the socio-economic status of women is notable in the light of the prevailing cultural circumstances in which women are subordinated in the society. This socio-economic deficiency make them to be excluded from participation in effective decisions that affect them, as well as make them dependent on men to take such decisions on matters of affecting their peculiar interest. Early studies has shown that the benefit of improve socio-economic status of women will not only help to improve the quality of life of women, but will also promote health and facilitate the social and political participation of women in matters that concern their health and lives.[197]

10.4.3. Expert views on Legislative Policy on Abortion and Contraception

There is a consensus among experts that legalizing abortion would lead to the increase in unwanted pregnancy among adolescent. Despite that, orthodox health expert believe liberalizing abortion would reduce drastically criminally complicated abortions and teenage maternal deaths. They held that orthodox health experts accused of breaching the law by perpetuating the practice do so first, for humanitarian reasons before the financial consideration. Researches have shown that, the appreciation and satisfaction received from helping others

---

[196] C. Nare, et al. 1997, Pp. 23.

[197] R. T. Bellew and E. M. King 1993, pp. 285.

(humanitarian) are the primary motivation of orthodox providers.[198] Dr. J. in an excerpt of interview stated it in this form,

> '...the doctors consider some of the negative implication on the lady (girl) .../ it would possibly lead the girl to stop school and terminate her educational career. She would lose affection of her parents. This could be traumatising. So doctors perpetuate it to save a lot of situations...the second consideration is the financial aspect which is not a reward, it is only a charge by the doctor for taking the risk of doing what the law considers as illegal...come to think of it, how much is the charge or pay when weighed against the risk? So you could see that the doctor is only assisting...'

The position of Dr. J. revealed that the appreciation and satisfaction received by orthodox practitioner from helping abortion victims is the motivation for many providers. They seem motivated in spite of the illegality, largely by psychic rewards of altruism and the enhanced social status of their position.[199]

Consequently, orthodox expert practitioners are of the view that government should liberalize abortion with some basic conditions. They held that this law was necessary in the light of illegally perpetuated abortions in spite of the law in public and private hospitals, traditional clinics, by quacks and other unorthodox practitioners. They outlined some of the benefits of the laws as,

- free treatment of adolescent victims and the poor who patronize quacks because of the high cost charged by orthodox clinics due to its illegality
- close monitoring of the activities of victims, and providers of such services, and
- help to reduce the high incidence of casualties resulting from death of both victims and child

Contrarily, unorthodox male experts argue that liberalizing or legalizing abortion is against tradition and the sanctity of life. They claim it would increase promiscuity among adolescents. The two female unorthodox experts disagreed with the position of their male counterparts. They believe that the law would help to reduce the spate of clandestine abortion and the deaths that results. One of them summed it up in this form,

> (Adi): ...legalizing abortion will prevent a lot of unwanted pregnancies... it would help to prevent deaths resulting from clandestine abortion-from both orthodox and unorthodox expert practitioners. Remember that abortion is illegal and yet most of us (I inclusive) and most other doctors in government hospitals still engaged in doing it illegally.../ I have to do it in spite, of the law because I need the money to feed my family; this is because it pays more since it is an illegal practice and the risk involved---

---

[198] James D. Shelton 2001, Pp. 152.
[199] Ibid 2001, Pp. 152-153

The concern expressed by the two female unorthodox practitioners was noteworthy and in line with those of the orthodox expert practitioners. However, the unorthodox male practitioners emphasize more on morality, ethics, tradition, religion and values to the detriment of the health and life of the girl child.

10.4.4. Legislative Concern

The staggering increase in deaths recorded in public hospitals due to the complications referred to it from illegal abortion of teenagers informed a bill initiated recently, by the Federal Ministry of Health, in concert with the Ministry of women Affairs and the Health Committee of the National Assembly in August 2001. The idea was to review the existing legislation on illegal abortion. Consultations was made by the head of the committee on Health in the National Assembly, Dr. beid with human right groups, women interest groups, prominent individual in order to articulate a comprehensive package before the second reading. In an excerpt of interview with Dr. beid he revealed the following,

> '...That the lack of consensus among women representatives themselves on such a sensitive issue is a cause for concern. Even women in the same political party and from other parties are divided among themselves...'

The above is an expression of doubts on the deliberation of the bill and the long time it would take for consensus to be reached by women themselves on such a crucial matter that affect them in Nigeria. Studies on Nepal women showed a similar trend where women are not united to fight a common cause that affect their health in terms of abortion law and other reproductive health matters.[200]

10.5. Conception of Respondents on Female Circumcision
10.5.1. Adolescent Views

Adolescents are divided in their views on female circumcision. During the focus group discussion and personal interview sessions, a total of sixteen out of seventeen adolescents were strongly opposed to the practice of female circumcision. Among the five adolescent males only one registered his support for the continuation of the practice. It is his position that the practice is a long held traditional and cultural one that must be continued. He insisted that he must circumcise his female children in the future because of the numerous advantages and benefits that he learned of the practice from his father, like sexual responsibility of circumcised women and enhancement of fertility.[201] His view are represented in the excerpt below,

> (I):   how do you see the practice of female circumcision?
>
> (KO): It is a good thing to do. I want girls to be circumcised. It makes them sexually responsible,

---

[200] Thapa Shyam and Padhye M. Saraswati 2001, Pp. 114

[201] Jane N. Chege, Ian Askew and Jennifer Liku 2001, Pp. 10-11.

not promiscuous. Because you as a man can travel and be sure that your wife won't be engaged in sexual acts on your behalf unlike uncircumcised women who can not control their urge for sex...

(I):   who told you what you know?

(KO):   my father told me that it is one of our tradition and culture that must be kept alive...women that are circumcised are also very fertile and give birth easily...I won't fail to circumcise all my female children in the future. I have personally experienced the circumcision of my two elder sisters...

In consensus the other four adolescent males condemn the practice and oppose it in its totality. They advocate that it be banned because of the health implication later in life on the girl. They claimed to have known about the health implications from either the experiences of their sisters or from what they had read in the books, magazines etc. They were of the opinion that the practice has no known advantages and that it is sustained for cultural purposes during which people gather to enjoy the gifts and good food cooked during the exercise to the detriment of the pains underwent by the female victim. This point shows that female circumcision is encouraged because the custom is believed to provide an important social and economic role for the practicing communities.[202] This point was explicit in the views of the proponents of female circumcision as revealed in the excerpt below,

(KO):   ...more so, after the circumcision of my sisters, they were well taken care off by my father's wives, who bathed and treated them well during the period...it was a time when very good meals and food was prepared for the entire household. You really enjoy this period in my home...

(I):   so it is because of the food---

(KO):   (cut in), not exactly, but that is just the way it is. Tradition must take its course...

Adolescent female were unanimous in their opposition to the practice. The twelve of them condemned the practice as barbaric and unhealthy to the health of the woman irrespective of their religious and ethnic inclinations. Only three of them were not circumcised because they hail from Itsekiri ethnic group where female circumcision is culturally disallowed. The others had gone through the surgical blades and knives of both traditional and orthodox health providers, as corroborated in earlier researches of Fran Hosken.[203]

Many of the adolescent females insist that they would enlighten their husbands in the future on the health hazards of the practice in order to prevent a similar

---

[202] Families in the Sabot tribe in Kenya, receive Cows upon the circumcision of their first girl. Such gifts are thought to be an economic basis for the girl to start life (Time, Dec. 3, 2001: 71) In most practicing communities in Nigeria, such gifts are shared by the girl and the family members

[203] Fran P. Hosken 1989, Pp. 3-6.

experience on their female children. However, they pointed out that if their husband insisted on the act on their female child and such threaten their marital home, they would have no alternative but to yield to their husband pressure in order to protect their home, family and marital relationship. Surprisingly, even those whose culture abhors the practice share a similar sentiment with the above view. This means that reproductive choice is a function of the 'male culture' of the Urhobo, Isoko and Okpe societies, which determines male and female status and power relationships in society. Thus the culture plays a role in the distribution of duties and responsibilities within the society. In this context, within marriage, men (husbands) and women (wives) have sexual, economic, domestic and other duties which are to a large extent culturally determined most of these roles and responsibilities are seen as properly belonging to the husband or men.[204] The gender implication is that the decision to continue or discontinue female circumcision in the Urhobo, Isoko and Okpe societies is rested more on the males because the practice is still deeply rooted in patrilineal and patrilocal social structure. Again, this emphasizes the traditional superiority of males over females. More so, the importance attached to marriage and the lower socio-economic status of women are inhibitive factors that affect the psychology of women in taking decisions on matters in which they are most affected. From gender perspective, female circumcision is not only a health problem but also, a combination of socio-economic, cultural and developmental problem.[205]

10.5.2. Adult views on Female Circumcision

Opinion on female circumcision varied among the adults. However, there was no gender difference among younger adults (20-39 years) and older adults (40 years and above) opinion and disposition to the discontinuation or continuation respectively, on the practice of female circumcision in the Urhobo, Okpe, Agbor, Isoko and other practicing communities in Delta state.

Older adult argue that female circumcision has a number of advantages such as, curbing promiscuity, enhancing neatness of the vagina, easing fertility, making the woman looks younger, beautifying the vagina region, make the woman matured und increases the marriage value and opportunity of the woman. They also claim that it is a form of cultural identity that should not be taken away under the guise of western cultural value judgement. It is their view that discouraging female circumcision is a form of interference by Western culture on tradition. Their view is congruent with those of Germaine Greer and Nosa Omoigui who called it another form of 'cultural imperialism' under the guise of globalisation of culture.[206]

Gender wise, female adults from the Urhobo, Okpe, and Isoko speaking areas expressed no regrets for undergoing the practice of female circumcision. They

---

[204] Carla Makhlouf Obermeyer 1994, Pp. 41-43.
[205] Margaret Brady 1999, Pp. 711-714.
[206] Germaine Greer 1999, Pp. 102 and Nowa Omoigui 2001, Pp. 8.

felt proud about it, and saw it as a symbol of women power and status; and even threatened to circumcise their granddaughters if their parents failed to carry out the traditional symbolic act of womanhood on them. The adult males share the worldview of the female adults for the continuation of the practice as highlighted above. In this context, female adults are the opinion leaders of the practice.

Younger adults do not share the position of the older adults. In particular, female victims in this category swore not to see their daughter go through the painful and traumatic experience. This category of adults, emphasize the health implications of the practice and called for an outright ban. Although, most of them would be prepared to give up their stand when it threatens their marital home. They also, recommended enlightenment campaign and programs to awaken the consciousness of pro-female circumcision advocates to understand the inherent dangers and emphasis on the right of the individual to protect their body from any form of harmful traditional and superstitious practices.[207]

10.5.3. Expert views on Female Circumcision

During the personal interview, opinions were divergent among specialists on female circumcision. The three expert practitioners were uniform in their responses that female circumcision is a 'mutilation of the female genitalia.' They hold that the practice is a dangerous and unhealthy traditional habit. Many researches have documented the many health dangers of this practice.[208] This position is appreciated clearly in the excerpt of interview with Mrs. Bea.

> ...female circumcision could leave a permanent scar after healing which is dangerous to the health of the woman in future when she starts having babies...the healed scar can re-tear and result in bleeding, contamination and even infections...

Another orthodox health expert practitioner enthused in the interview as revealed below,

> (Dr. J): ...I do not see any advantages in female circumcision...it is just a cultural and traditional practice...uncircumcised women may not be 'over sexually sensitive' as been portrayed by traditionalist. The belief that women must be circumcised before giving birth in most communities or else the babies would die has been proved to be medically wrong...

The responses indicate that orthodox health expert practitioners view the practice of female circumcision as medically unhealthy, and they advocate an attitudinal change through education and enlightenment campaigns in communities where the practice is still deeply entrenched, and in the meantime, they recommend a medicalized approach until an appropriate law was promulgated to ban the

---

[207] D. R. McCaffery 1995, Pp. 790.

[208] M. A. Dirie and G. Lindmark 1992, Pp. 479-482, / U. Linke 1986, Pp. 203 and Nahid Toubia 1995, Pp. 4.

practice.[209] They blamed parents who at these times of modernity still subject their daughters to such harmful traditional practice. Worse still, they condemned trado-medical midwives, herbalist and native doctors for carrying out the act or operation. In the same vein they accused and laid blames on some of their colleagues who engage in the act just for the financial benefit even with their medical knowledge of the health hazards and implications.

Unorthodox health expert practitioners are on the side of tradition and the continuation of the practice. The four of them interviewed (2 males and 2 females) were openly or tacitly in support of the practice for one reason or the other. The female practitioners agreed to have been involved in the circumcision of females at one time or the other during their practice as traditional reproductive health providers. Though they agreed that the process was very painful, but not enough for one to advocate its outright ban. They recommend that the process of circumcision be medicalised to ease the pains with modern medicine. One of them described the process she adopted in circumcising females about five years ago in this form,

> (Mak): ... the time I did female circumcision was a very long time ago. I used razor blade and scissors...what I do is that a strong man was made to sit at the breast level of the girl to hold her tightly to the ground while I did the cutting of a part of the clitoris that could make the girl sexually too sensitive. After the operation I applied a very hot substance from mixture of traditional herbs and share cropping latex to the open wound, this application is very hot and painful and it help to kill the sore...I have stopped doing this, since about 5 years now. I personally passed through the same process, but this was some years ago. Now there are easy ways to do it with modern medicines without the girl feeling any much pain. This is done by nurses in the hospital...so, they could use the modern approach and not to cancel the practice...

When asked why she stopped the practiced, she claimed to have sourced other avenue of earning income at old age, instead of getting money that comes through painful and very demanding exercise like female circumcision.

The other female traditional midwife agreed with the above position of Madam Mak, that it is a source of her own income. To her it is the major reason why she carries out the practice and not because there is any known advantages even though she underwent the same process when she was younger. The excerpt reveals further,

> (Adi): there are no clear gains of female circumcision... however an uncircumcised female has more feeling of sex than the circumcised one. On the other hand, a circumcised woman could suffer vagina tear during childbirth and without adequate care she could bleed to death. This is not

---

[209] Karen Engle 1992, Pp. 1115.

> common with uncircumcised women. So both have their advantages and disadvantages... in fact, if government is to outlaw it, it is only going to affect one major source of my income. But to be quite frank, circumcised women are more in danger of losing their lives during childbirth because of the risk of tear...I know this and I have experienced this in my practice...

The above views reveal a lot on the practice of female circumcision. The sincerity of the cultural reasons given for the perpetuation of the practice is thus questionable when viewed against the economic reasons that underlie the aims and purpose of traditional midwives and practitioners.

Unorthodox expert male practitioners are strongly in favour of the practice. They hold that it is a practice that has helped to curb the decadence of sexual promiscuity and the reduction of sexual urges among women; and that this has helped to sanitize the moral basis of society by controlling the spate of adultery among women. They claimed not to have been involved in circumcision as part of their practice but have ensured that all their female children and wives have gone through the process of female circumcision as a 'cultural necessity.' They call for the preservation of the act and for government to improve the process of the exercise with modern medical technology rather than advocate for the extinction of an important aspect of the peoples culture.[210]

10.6. Conception of Respondents on Legislative Policy on Female Circumcision

10.6.1. Adolescent Views

Seventeen adolescents but one advocate an effective legislative policy by both state and federal government to ban female circumcision as a harmful traditional practice. One of the adolescent female encapsulated it in this form,

> (Miss OK): ...passing or making the laws to ban this crude act is one thing and implementing such a law is another...some states claim to have outlawed the practice, but it is still secretly done. This is Nigeria for you...

The position of doubt expressed by Miss OK is understood in the context of law implementation in Nigeria. The sixteen adolescents in consensus agreed that with an effective law in place, parents, husbands, traditional midwives and community leaders would be deterred from embarking on this act under the guise of social pressure, horror trip, economic benefits etc. used as reasons to perpetuate the practice of female circumcision. It is their conception that an effective legislation should begin with an awareness campaign to highlight the dangers of the practice in all cultural practicing communities in Nigeria. In supporting a strong awareness and educational campaign, early research studies states "that circumcision principal purpose is to make its victims incapable of

---

[210] Ibid, 1992, Pp. 1515

sexual feelings and there is the need to devote efforts to national organization for women to raise awareness and generate support for anti-female circumcision movements."[211] One of the adolescent male discussant portrayed it in the form below,

> (Okev): The government knows what to do to make any law banning female circumcision effective/…but they are accomplices in such cases------/ my position remain that any such law should start with enlightening every individual of the dangers of female circumcision----so, on the on-going campaign parents, community leaders and women should be targeted…

Women are regarded as conspirators and accomplices from the obvious position of the above opinions. For instance, most of the adolescent females who had gone through the surgical knives and razor blades were taken to the spot where the act was, carried out on them by their mothers, sisters, or grand mothers. Studies in Kenya, and Somalia has also revealed that women who had undergone the process often wanted it done on their female children either now or in the future.[212]

Adolescents advocate an effective legislation that would enable them to have the right to choose if they wanted the act to be performed on them or not. Studies showed an existing law promulgated in 1997 in the United States that makes it an offence for a child of under 18 years to be circumcised. Though the law did not cover women over 18 years old, but the important thing was that it created an avenue for female choice at that age.[213]

Adolescents held that such a law banning the practice would help to prevent parents and even traditional advocate from carrying out such acts that terrorises and threaten their health by capitalizing on their innocence. Parents and traditionalists have adopted, deception, threat, horror trip, social pressures, gift giving to woe females to circumcise, particularly among the Urhobo and Okpe ethnic groups. Miss Adib reports her experience below,

> 'the day my parents reached a decision on my circumcision I suspected because my elder sister had given me a clue some days before…I was very scared but on the actual day, it was my mother that took me by hand to the place----I did not suspect until I got there…'

This suggest that parents adopt 'tacit deceit' to lure their children to perpetuate the act. Miss Adib would have suspected the move of her parents if both of them had accompanied her on the said day to the traditional midwife and probably, she would have defected or resisted. There are many other variant to this deceptive

---

[211] William Raspberry 1993, Pp. A21
[212] DHS 1995, Pp. 173.
[213] Margaret Brady 1999, Pp. 715.

strategies adopted by parents as shown by studies on 'alternative rights approach for encouraging abandonment of female genital mutilation in Kenya.'[214]

Only one male in this category was opposed to the law banning female circumcision. He decries any such legislation on traditional and cultural ground, and the benefits of the practice to the male folk.

10.6.2. Adult views on Legislative Policy On Female Circumcision

Younger adults (20-34 years) maintained that the practice of female circumcision is bad and call for an effective legislation to ban the practice and check the perpetrators of it. They further advocate a pre-enlightenment campaign to be organized by government in concert with the federal and state ministries of health, in corporation with Non Governmental agencies (NGOs), human rights groups, women organizations etc. to sensitise various communities and culture groups, and opinion leaders on the health implications of the practice. They held that change agents should incorporate local organisations otherwise it would, be seen as harbouring a colonialist agenda.[215]

The incorporation of local organizations would help to disabuse the minds of practicing communities that government intention is aim at interfering with age long tradition, and deriding of the peoples culture. The emphasis here is on craving the *understanding* of the health hazard of female circumcision and the need to improve the health of the girl child as well as understanding the socio-cultural context in which the practice exist[216], and help to erase the impression that it is another western form of 'cultural imperialism' or intervention of cultural sovereignty of the people.

Older adults on their part expressed negative attitude towards any legislation to ban female circumcision. They drew attention to the traditional basis for their argument. They also expressed socio-cultural and political fears that their culture would fade away in the interest of western cultural imperialist.

According to Madam Mak:

> ' as for me, an Urhobo woman, I strongly want (angrily) both men and particularly, women to be circumcised, that is our culture, it is our tradition.../ and we must not let it die because of a few educated people who want to adopt the white man's culture...our own is our own...'

The impression above was that of an expressed gender objection to the ban of female circumcision in practicing Urhobo and Okpe ethnic groups for 'fear of cultural imperialism.' Some Nigerian feminist writers argues in favour of this point, that it is an intervention of western idea on a progressive indigenous culture by redefining female circumcision in terms of 'genital mutilation' thereby

---

[214] Jane N. Chege, Ian Askew and Jennifer Liku 2001, Pp. 12-32.

[215] MFAD 1995, Pp. 17

[216] Seble Dawit and Salem Mekuria 1993, Pp. 27.

112

making it sound crude and dangerous.[217] This political colouration is an abuse of the indigenous cultures right to practice their cherished tradition. This was further, amplified by an adult male who claimed thus,

> (Jon): if the issue is in terms of death resulting from the crude method of circumcision of females as claimed, then government should help us to improve on the operational process rather than asking us to throw away our tradition and culture...

The older adults are firm in their resolve that government is trying to compromise with western interests to extinct their valuable traditional practice and rather called for the medicalization of the practice. Hence the younger adults request a proper enlightenment campaign in this direction since all segment of society both old and young perceive that the practice could be dangerous if not properly managed. This is put in Mrs Egbo words in the form beneath,

> 'there is a common ground between supporters and oppositionist on banning female circumcision. We all agree that the practice is hazardous, whether it is well done or not to the health of the woman, what should be done now, is to work out the method of cooperation and the only way out is through awareness campaigns and enlightenment of the people before the law is promulgated------'

There is no contention with regards to the dangers of female circumcision but the main area of altercation is in the area of the method to be adopted in ameliorating or avoiding these health hazards.[218]

10.6.3. Expert views on the Legislative Policy on Female Circumcision

The experts are in consensus that female circumcision could result in health problems. But while orthodox health experts held that the health complications manifest from the day the girl child was circumcised, the unorthodox health experts believe that such health complications only results when 'the act was not well performed.' The orthodox health experts are unequivocal in their call for a law to ban the practice, and they recommend that such a law should be referred to as the 'female circumcision act.' They also advice that government should embark on pre-enlightenment campaigns of practicing communities to understand the purpose for such act rather than see it as a way of culture cleansing.[219] Dr. J. summed up the position of the orthodox health experts as follows,

> '...a law to ban female circumcision would be welcome. It would be fine. I support government totally. But beyond that government should try and educate the multiplicity of ethnic communities to understand the dangers inherent in the practice.

---

[217] Nowa Omoigui 2001, Pp. 8
[218] Karen Engle 1992, Pp. 1516.
[219] Jane N. Chege, et al. 2001, Pp. 38

> They should *not adopt the use of force in*
> *enlightening* cultural groups. Remember culture
> change is supposed to be gradual.../ government
> should do a lot of persuasion and convincing...

The watchword in the position of orthodox health experts is 'persuasive reasoning' and not the 'use of forceful language' that would raise the emotions and feelings of practicing communities in the direction of suspicion of 'cultural imperialism or cultural extinction.' More so, a forceful legislation may drive the practicing communities of Urhobo, Okpe, Bini, Isoko and individuals to engage in the act secretly and underground, and this may spell more danger to the health of women.[220]

Orthodox health experts called for both international and local support beyond the local legislation to fight this source of health hazard on women. This is encapsulated in Mrs Bea, words as follows,

> '...Obviously it will take more than just legislation
> to eradicate this practice that can no longer be seen
> as religious or traditional custom/...one cannot
> mount an ethical defence for a practice that result
> in such negative impacts on a woman's health. This
> is not only a problem for countries like Nigeria
> where it is performed but also for the western
> world...

This suggests how difficult the struggle to embark on the campaign against the practice of female circumcision is when localized strictly; particularly, in deep - rooted traditional societies. The need for collective resource materials and manpower to confront the issue is emphasized. This validates the positions of Mary Brady and Egan in their work on, 'Female Genital Mutilation: Complications and the Risk of HIV Transmission' and their call that opponent of female circumcision should ultimately seek the assistance of international legislation and education to help eradicate the practice.[221]

The unorthodox health experts argue on their part that the law banning female circumcision is not necessary as the practice is still very widely accepted by the people and performs the function of helping to integrate the woman into various structures and institutions of the community where it is practiced like the marriage institution, and the right of passage to womanhood and even curbing promiscuity. It was their opinion that the advantages of the practice is so immense, that it would amount to 'cultural suicide' to out law it. Madam Mak expressed it in the following interview excerpt,

> '...Many here in my community dispute claims that
> there is any health risk associated with the age long
> practice...female circumcision has no negative
> effects as claimed by modern medicine, if that is the
> problem, then let them use the modern medicine to

---

[220] MFAD 1995, Pp. 17.
[221] Margaret Brady 1999, Pp. 715-716 / T. Egan 1993, Pp. A25

> improve the operation instead of trying to do away with a practice that performs a great role for society and the woman...'

The need to medicalize the procedure of operation was proposed by this traditional school of thought, rather than tamper with culture. The same opinion was canvass by unorthodox male expert. For Chief Jon, he conceptualised it in this form,

> '...God forbid that female circumcision be banned, this ruling cannot work in this our community...it would definitely continue in secret...'

This declaration by Chief Jon is an indication of the difficulty that would be encountered if a proper awareness structure are not in place to educate the people on the need for the reverse thinking and practice of female circumcision even if the law was promulgated.

The unorthodox health experts also listed what they consider as the advantages of female circumcision as follows, reduces feelings of unnecessary sexual arousal in women, make them less likely to engage in pre-marital sex and consequently, cannot be victims of the crime of adultery, make them find marriage partners easily, clitoris is dangerous to the woman's health if not removed, clitoris is poisonous to the male organ if not removed, it can make the man to fall ill and even die, it eliminates bad genital odours, prevents vagina diseases or cancer, prevents self masturbation or lesbianism practice by women, makes the woman to always look younger and beautiful, enhances fertility of the woman, make the man to be able to match the woman sex drives unlike an uncircumcised woman, and it makes the woman not to be infected with diseases easily. All of these reasons have been mentioned in one form or the other in earlier researches.[222]

Some of the reasons given have been criticized by feminist advocates to be more gender sensitive for male oriented satisfaction, to keep sustaining the practice.[223] But the unorthodox health experts from the Urhobo, and Okpe ethnic groups presume it to play a functional role in the regulation of social order in such communities where it is deeply rooted. Noteworthy, is the opposition raised by an unorthodox female health expert to the views of her colleagues. Mrs Adi contend that the practice is deadly and that she perpetuates it to earn income in her trade. Her views are further expressed below,

> '...to be very frank, I support government proposal to ban female circumcision because the delivery of the uncircumcised women are very free unlike the circumcised woman----/ and most women in order to defend themselves from the feeling of inferiority, deny that female circumcision damages their bodies or sexuality...'

---

[222] Olayinka Koso-Thomas 1987, Pp. 1-3
[223] A. M. Rosenthal 1993, Pp. 15-33.

From a gender construct, Mrs. Adis contention challenges the position of old generation or adult women who claim that female circumcision is a test for a 'real woman'. She holds that the introduction of deception and 'self obfuscation' as strategies by women to convince their daughters or girls to have them circumcised is not in the best interest of women if the practice is to be discouraged.

Thus many 'anti- female circumcision advocates' especially the adolescents, younger adults and the orthodox health experts suggest that the legislation to ban female circumcision must take into consideration all shed of opinions and target principally, women in the enlightenment campaigns as they sometimes form the resistant bracket in their own affairs.[224] Mrs Okpa summed it up in following way,

> '...if any legislation is to be effective, most women should be made to develop the sensitivity to feel deprived or to see in female circumcision practice a violation of their human rights...this is the only way out. We should first as women try to help ourselves...'

The above position exposes the socio-cultural, economic and educational deprivation of women in the larger society that impede their conceptualisation and understanding of their rights on matters that affects them.[225]

---

[224] Seble Dawit and Salem Mekuria 1993, Pp. 27.
[225] Elspeth Probyn 1992, Pp. 83.

11.0. Chapter eleven
Discourse Analysis of stated Hypotheses on Abortion and Female Circumcision
11.1. Discourse analysis of stated hypotheses on abortion
This section discusses analytically the five (5) stated hypotheses in section 1.5.1. (1). Adolescent females engage in the use of illegal abortion to terminate unwanted pregnancies.
Discourse
To discuss the above stated hypothesis, the views of the forty-four (44) respondents or participants was analysed and they all hold the same position as stated in the hypothesis. However, they attributed varied reasons for that. Orthodox health experts attribute the reason to the law banning abortion in Nigeria except to save the life of the woman, as the reason why adolescent seek alternative and dangerous channels to get rid of unwanted pregnancies. Adolescents themselves attribute the reasons to the fear of apprehension by law enforcement agents as deterrent from procuring abortion within the limit of the law in public and privately established clinics and hospitals. Some others, claim ignorance of the law on adolescent health matters, lack of money, lack of the courage to buy protective pills or condoms and other 'over-the counter' devices, as well as peer group influences and pressures for seeking and engaging in the use of illegal abortion to terminate unwanted pregnancies. These views were consistent with the findings of Shyam and Saraswati in their studies of 'induced abortion in Urban Nepal' where abortion is severely restricted by law, thus prompting women seeking abortions and most people providing abortion services to do so illegally and clandestinely.[226]

Adults attribute the breakdown in the values of tradition to adolescent behaviour in resorting to the adoption of illegal abortion. To them, some part of the society have undergone change in values towards permissiveness for teenage pregnancies, and that most parents are rather pursuing material survival to the detriment of instilling discipline and control on their children. They also impress on western value influences like education, the technological aspects like the Television, Films, Video, Print and other forms of electronic media, which are used to transmit obscene pictures and immoral scenes in the name of advertisements.

All participant especially, adolescent respondents accepted to have *heard, known* and *experienced* directly or indirectly, situations where adolescent female have been victims of illegal abortion to get rid of unwanted pregnancies or attempted at it. This is consistent with the findings of the joint research of the Kenya National Council for Population and the John Hopkins University Communication Services on 'Reproductive Health Communication in Kenya' in August and September 1994. Even the orthodox health experts holds, that the

---

[226] Thapa Shyam and Padhye M. Saraswati 2001, Pp. 144.

117

large number of deaths that result which often go unrecorded is an attestation and validation of the adoption of illegal abortion by adolescent females. In fact, what is known about women seeking pregnancy termination in countries with restrictive laws has been learned from women admitted into hospitals with abortion related complications. Little is known about women who obtain 'safe' abortions from trained providers.[227]

Participants mentioned the various methods and individuals, used and implicated for the perpetuation of illegal abortion to include, self-medication of drugs, consultation with quacks- like chemist operators, traditional herbalist and midwives, auxiliary nurses, and even some orthodox expert health providers etc.

Advocates of legalization or liberalisation of abortion argue that such a law may not only be very relevant to resolving the problems of unwanted pregnancy among adolescent females, but also primarily help to control family size and birth spacing in Nigeria and decrease tremendously the numbers of illegally perpetuated abortions, especially those that are of high risk and unsafe.[228]

(2). That adolescent females rely on the use of ineffective contraceptives to prevent and induce unwanted pregnancies.

Discourse

As a corollary to the first discussed hypothesis, all forty-four (44) participants were concerted in their opinion. Participants mentioned various forms of ineffective contraceptives applied by adolescents. Most of these contraceptives were found to be crude and dangerous, and are made up of combinations of modern and traditional herbs. For instance there is the mention of mixed herbal materials inserted into the vagina of the girl to cause bleeding; the mixture of local gin with M and B tablets or Codeine tablet for the girl to drink, the self medication of drugs like Prostinol, Menstrogen, and the mixture of Potash, and lime juice for the girl to drink, mixture of tetracycline capsules with gin or stout for the girl to drink etc. All these were acknowledged to be highly corrosive and dangerous. While others were said to apply the use of the latex from boundary (see Appendix VI-16) into the vagina of the girl, and still others, given a combination of un-prescribed injections.

There was a consensus on the part of the adolescents, orthodox health experts and younger adult respondents, that adolescents resort to the use of ineffective Contraceptives because of the law banning abortion and their limited access to contraceptives usage, couple with the peer group influences, poor knowledge of sex education, poverty and timidity on their part. Striking similarities with the

---

[227] Ibid 2001, Pp.144
[228] International Family Planning Perspectives (IFPP) 2001, Vol. 27 (3), Pp. 144-151.

above, have been expressed in previous studies on health of adolescents in Nigeria.[229]

Older adults and unorthodox health experts blame all of these situations on the breakdown of traditional values as well as western cultural influences, and more importantly on the ineffective implementation of the law banning abortion.

There was no contention among all forty-four participants on the views expressed except in the area of laying blames or responsibility on whom, was the greatest accomplices in the act of perpetuating illegal abortion, between the orthodox and unorthodox health experts. It was also clear that in spite, of the contention between both parties, they were both implicated as culprits in performing illegal abortion for financial and humanitarian reasons. Previous study on abortion holds that the lack of review of the existing abortion law is the major cause of this trend. The study reveal that this has led to the obscurity of the quality of services provided by both orthodox and unorthodox health experts, and that under such conditions, health care providers generally deny their involvement in or practice of illegal abortion. This may have contributed to the ambiguity stated during the discussion by some of the adolescents in accessing a competent abortion care provider.[230]

(3). That adolescents have restricted access to safe contraception
Discourse
Orthodox health experts holds that the increase in spate of illegal abortions and the use of ineffective contraceptives to prevent and induce unwanted pregnancies by adolescents are propelled by the law restricting abortions and the limited access to Contraceptives. Also, it is their conception that the restriction placed on the consultation of the few available and existing family planning units and ante-natal clinics was bound to encourage the use of unsafe contraception by adolescents.

Adolescents hold that because of their ignorance and lack of information on health matters, they are unaware of services provided by existing health care units like the Family planning and the ante-natal care units of public health institutions in Sapele, Jesse and Oghare-efe. Adolescents from Sapele, Jesse and Oghare-efe agreed that they rely on secondary sources of information that are informal like hear-says, peer group influences, friends or indirect experiences of others. Even the few that were knowledgeable claim to be afraid to consult such existing health provision clinics because of the existing law that does not only restrict abortions but also exclude adolescent in their considerations. Consequently, adolescents resort to unsafe contraception when the need arose. Thus adolescents do not feel that having to obtain Contraceptives was a major

---

[229] Friday E. Okonofua, et al. 1999, Pp.184-190 /Valentine Otoide, et al. 2001, Pp. 79-81

[230] F. Olowu 1998, Pp. 49-60.

hindrance to use, contrary to findings from several published studies.[231] Consequently, adolescent felt that the restrictive law in place against abortion and access to Contraceptives endears them to the easy access and services of patent medicine dealers and most times unorthodox health experts who were to them sufficient to meet their contraceptive needs, as these providers are located within reach on street corners and surprisingly they provide confidential services. This also explained adolescent knowledge and use of modern antibiotics and other medications, as contraceptives as these likely were recommended and procured from patent medicine dealer as well as from unorthodox health experts.[232] Previous studies have shown these categories of service providers often are not trained and have diverse educational backgrounds with a significant number of them not literate.[233]

Older adults and unorthodox health experts held contrary views from those of the adolescents and orthodox health experts. They argued that adolescents should not be exposed to safe contraception in order not to increase the spate of indiscriminate sex and a breakdown of societal values of sex value and sanctity. Rather, they advocate strict parental control on children, inculcation of traditional and religious moral values on teenagers, improvement of the social economic status of women through provision of adequate education, to enable them gain good employment and become economically independent and be able to take control of all tempting sexual attractions for monetary reasons, and effective implementation of government laws banning abortion and strict access to Contraceptives. However, there was no contention among all shed of participants or respondents that adolescents would resort to unsafe Contraception when faced with limited choices on what to do about an unwanted pregnancy.

(4). That many adolescents are unaware of the abortion law in Nigeria
Discourse
When asked if they (adolescents) were aware if abortion is legal or illegal? They responded uniformly -that abortion is illegal. When further asked to state what they knew about the law on abortion, they could not. They were also not able to state or even furnish the source of their information beyond giving religious (Christian) reasons and other informal sources such as traditional sanctions, and parental teaching etc. Only two adolescent females claimed to have read about

---

[231] C. Nare, K. Kate and E. Tolley 'Adolescents access to reproductive health and family planning services in Dakar (Senegal)', *African Journal of Reproductive Health*, 1997, 1(2): 15-24; and F. Olowu 'Quality and Cost of Family Planning as elicited by an adolescent mystery client trial in Nigeria', African Journal of Reproductive Health, 1998, 12(1): 49-60.

[232] Valentine Otoide, et al. 2001, Pp. 80.

[233] Friday E. Okonofua et al, 'Assessment of health services for treatment of sexually transmitted infections among Nigerian adolescents', *Sexually Transmitted Diseases*, 1999, 26(3): 184-190

the laws on abortion from the books, but could not effectively articulate the laws when asked to do so.

More so, even the adults and unorthodox health experts could not state the laws, even when they claimed adequate knowledge of it. They also claimed their source of knowledge from both modern Christian, Islamic and traditional religions that condemns the shedding of blood as a sin and against God, and the gods of the land.

This vacuum in the knowledge and awareness of abortion law by respondents or participants is upheld as one the greatest problems of reproductive health care in Nigeria. Recent studies have exposed the ignorance of adolescents on the abortion law and contraceptive usage. They argued that the lack of adolescent knowledge and understanding of the laws on abortion makes them very vulnerable in the hands of quacks and unorthodox health providers, and that it also, lead to adolescent adoption of methods ineffective in preventing unwanted pregnancies.[234] They believe that adequate information about the law on abortion, and knowledge of the use of contraceptives will be important in adolescent acceptance of modern methods of contraceptives, and their use of such methods at first intercourse.

(5). That adolescents advocate liberalization or legalization of abortion in Nigeria

Discourse

To evaluate the above hypothesis adolescents were asked their views on liberalizing abortion laws. Thirteen out of seventeen adolescents suggested liberalization of the law. They gave reasons variedly for their suggestions, such as:

- all girls can have access to abortion irrespective of whether she is from a rich or poor background
- improve the health of women
- reduce the death of teenage mothers through illegal abortion
- reduce consultation with quacks
- reduce the costs implication of procuring illegal abortion on the part of the victim and government
- reduce the application of self medication of dangerous combination of drugs on the part of the victim
- sanitize society from the 'unwanted baby saga' that causes menace to the society.

In confirming the position of this pro-liberalization advocate who constitutes about 79.4 percent of adolescents. Some researchers have argued that, without a liberalized access to the abortion and contraceptives services, only a small percentage of women, mostly those from better socio-economic conditions and

---

[234] Frank Oronsaye, et al. 2001, Pp. 80.

backgrounds, will have access to safe abortions services; and other women will likely have no choice but to submit to the inherently high-risk and high-priced clandestine abortions.[235] Only Four other adolescents (all females) do not favour a policy of liberalization on abortion. They hinged their views on religious and moral principles, like the biblical injunction quoted in Exodus 20 verse 13 that 'thou shall not kill'. Still others believe that such a law would increase the level of sexual immorality in the society. These objecting adolescent females constitute about 20.6 per cent of the total adolescents. They also condemn outright the provision of young people with free contraceptives or free access to it. The oppositionist position is summed up from a religious perspective that, "every persons body is a gift, a stewardship, from God, and that the body is not meant for sexual immorality, but for the Lord, and the Lord for the body and that the control of one's body is not a moral right, but a moral responsibility, and that personal rights end when exercise of them could or does lead to endangering one's own life or the lives of others e.g. drunk driving and drug addiction; murder...endangering another's life through negligence...In abortion, it is the status of these 'others'- the unborn." [236]

However, the adolescent protagonist of liberalization of abortion hold that any such law on abortion should be accompanied by laid down conditions and standard in order, to avoid abuse of the process by victims and perpetrators.

Adolescents recommend effective sex education for all young people before the age of puberty when they are more sexually active. Such effective education they argued, will lead to attitudinal change towards reckless sex and the inherent dangers.

The orthodox health experts supported the position of adolescent protagonist for a liberalized law, even when they argue that liberalization of the law on abortion would lead to increase in unwanted pregnancy, but that it would also help to reduce significantly the tendency of teenage maternal deaths resulting from illegal and criminal abortion. The unorthodox health experts toe the argument of adolescent antagonists on the liberalization of abortion. They argue, that for the sake of religious, traditional and cultural values of morality and sanctity of life that abhor killing amongst many cultural and traditional groups like the Urhobo, Okpe, Isoko, Iteskiri and Bini ethnic groups, under any guise, liberalization of abortion should be discouraged. However, orthodox health experts held that since the Nigerian law prohibits abortion, the services provided are generally of poor and dangerous quality, which endangers the health of female adolescent victims. Similar trend was revealed in findings on a research conducted on 'adolescent reproductive behaviour' in Benin City, Nigeria.[237]

---

[235] Thapa Shyam and Padhye M. Saraswati 2001, Pp. 147.
[236] Randy Alcorn 1992, Pp. 1-4.
[237] Valentine Otoide, et al. 2001, Pp. 80.

11.2. Discourse analysis of stated hypotheses on female circumcision

This section discusses analytically the eight stated hypotheses on female circumcision.

11.2.a. Cultural Hypotheses on Female Circumcision

(1). That female circumcision enhances women fertility.

Discourse

One of the commonest reasons given for the legitimisation of female circumcision in Urhobo, Okpe, Isoko, and Bini practicing communities is that culturally, female circumcision enhances fertility of the woman. To verify this claim, orthodox and unorthodox expert health providers were asked during the interview if the assertion was correct. The three orthodox health experts stated that though 'fertility can be sometimes culturally related in traditional societies, it was more a biological and medical issue.' The orthodox health experts emphatically stated, that there are rather serious obstetrical complications arising from female circumcisions that could result in infertility of the woman. Medical researches confirmed the position of orthodox health experts that, among all other complications mentioned, a long- term effect of female circumcision is sterility- another medical term for infertility.[238] Orthodox health experts listed areas of common grounds between circumcised and uncircumcised women which culture has no explanations except western and modern medical knowledge. They founded their clarification on the high points below that:

- there are women who are circumcised and are still barren
- there are women from communities that do not practice female circumcision like the Itsekiris, Tivs, Akwa- Ibomites, Oturkpo, and some part of Ika speaking peoples in Nigeria that are very fertile and gave birth to living children
- there are cases of uncircumcised women from practicing communities that have been found in hospital records to have gave birth to more than one surviving child
- the claim of fertility linked to the issue of female circumcision is a strategy to instil fear on their victims in order to sustain the practice,
- fertility issue is purely a complicated biological and medical issue that cannot be interpreted solely in terms of culture.

However, unorthodox health experts believe that female circumcision enhances the fertility chance of the woman except when the operation was not well done. Although, they could not sustain their claim with proofs of why some circumcised women from Jesse, Okpe, Urhobo and Isoko practicing communities were barren despite a well -done circumcision, and could also, not explain the fecundity of uncircumcised women in these same practicing communities. Their arguments were all based on traditional and cultural backgrounds.

---

[238] A. M. Rosenthal 1993c, Pp. 15.

Orthodox health experts observed and revealed that women from practicing ethnic groups like the Urhobo, Okpe, Isoko and Bini and non-practicing practicing ethnic groups like the Itsekiri, and Akwa-Ibom have been examined or treated for infertility at one point in time or the other during their medical practice. According to them, it was therefore, difficult to conclude on the claim of an existing relationship between female circumcision and the enhancement of women fertility from traditional and cultural conviction. Many early studies support the position of orthodox health experts on the danger of female circumcision on fertility of the woman. Ozumba (1992) and Rowe (1985) in their individual findings among circumcised women in Eastern Nigeria; and the world wide pattern of infertility respectively, pointed out that female circumcision could result in a common complication of sexually transmitted diseases known as the Pelvic Inflamatory Disease (PID) which is often accompanied by abdominal pains, infertility and ectopic pregnancy.[239] The estimated number of victims is put at about 22 and 44 percents of gynaecological cases in Africa hospitals. Calder, B. et al. (1993) amplified the point when he stated in his study, "female circumcision can result in obstetrical complications for the mother and foetus/baby."[240]

Scientific researcher also argue in support of orthodox health experts, that an estimated two to twenty-five per cent of cases of infertility in Sudan have been attributed to female circumcision in the form of infibulation, resulting either from chronic pelvic infection or because of the difficulty in having sexual intercourse and lack of penetration.[241]

(2). That female circumcision reduces sexual promiscuity on the part of the woman.

Discourse

The proponents of female circumcision especially among the Urhobo, Okpe and Isoko ethnic groups that I studied believe that the practice help to reduce the level or degree of promiscuity among women. The clitoris is believed to make the woman sexually excited, and that since she cannot control her sexual desires she becomes sexually immoral and cannot stick to one man. Thus control of sexual desire is a definition of true womanhood among the Urhobo, Okpe, Isoko and Bini speaking people. Therefore, excision is believed to protect a woman against her oversexed nature, saving her from temptation, suspicion and disgrace, while preserving her chastity. Culturally, 'not giving in' to sexual advances is considered honourable for a woman. This is similar to the reasons for the legitimisation of the practice among the Maasai, Meru, Abagusii and Kalenji ethinic groups of Kenya[242] and the Somali people.[243] However, studies have also

---

[239] P. J. Rowe 1985, Pp. 99 / B. C. Ozumba 1992, Pp. 105.
[240] B. Calder, et al. 1993, Pp. 712.
[241] Margaret Brady 1999, Pp. 712-713.
[242] Jane N. Chege, et al. 2001, Pp. 11.

revealed that female circumcision has not helped the issue of curbing promiscuity, particularly among the Maasai women in Kenya, the practice of female circumcision is a status symbol and symbol of women power, during the rite of passage into womanhood. In spite, of being circumcised the women still kept boy friends outside the matrimonial homes.[244]

Orthodox health experts also revealed significantly different argument from the positions of unorthodox health experts, and those of older adults from the Urhobo, Okpe, Isoko and Bini practicing communities. Orthodox health experts debunked the cultural belief that the clitoris has a correlation with sexual promiscuity of the woman. One of the respondents Dr. J stated 'that if there was a correlation between the clitoris and sexual promiscuity in practicing communities, they should explain in his words, the category of circumcised women in these same communities that are adulterous, and circumcised young girls who engage in rampant sex without protection in today's society'. The statement shows that even in practising communities adulterous women are seen as promiscuous and incidentally, these are the same women who underwent female circumcision. Tradition in this context, could only explain such cases as exceptional ones that is normal in any society, since there was nothing like a perfect system.

However, many recent medical and feminists studies have argued that, the uncut clitoris has no relationship with female promiscuity. The clitoris in such studies have been described medically and biologically to be responsible for pleasure and the enjoyment of sex. The studies explained further that, biologically, in all types of circumcision even the most 'mild' clitoridectomy (excision of the clitoris), a part of the woman's body contains nerves of vital importance to sexual enjoyment and if amputated, it causes a vital damage to the glands clitoridis with its specific sensory enjoyment at the primary erogenic zone. Furthermore, when it has been reduced to an area of scar tissue, no orgasm can be released by its manipulation. The well known William Masters and Viriginia Johnson, has conclusively proved that all orgasms in women originate in the clitoris, although they may be felt elsewhere.[245]

Studies have also pointed to the misunderstanding and confusion of practicing communities of the term 'stimulation' when the clitoris is uncut with 'sexual promiscuity'.[246] One of my female orthodox interviewee (Mrs. Bea), said, 'it was necessary for the woman to be stimulated before having sex because it help to lubricate the vagina before penetration and lessen pains on the woman. Circumcised women have been known to suffer frigidity and pains during sex and this make them not to enjoy sex to the benefit of the men.' This does not only make the sex experience painful and result in short and long-terms physical

---

[243] M. Arbesman, et al. 1993, Pp. 24 –25.
[244] Jane N. Chege, et al. 2001, Pp. 12.
[245] Scilla McLean 1980, Pp. 5.
[246] J. M. Irvine 1990, Pp. 162.

harms but it also manifest in mental, emotional and traumatic effects and experiences on the woman. Some researchers describe the psychological effects of Female circumcision as ranging from anxiety to severe depression and psychosomatic illnesses.[247]

Older adults contradicted their position when they could not reconcile the increase in indiscriminate sex among adolescent females in female circumcision practicing communities in Sapele, Jesse, and Oghara with the reality. Younger adults rather explained away the point by attributing the situation to the poor and changing socio-economic and political state of the country, like poverty as the propelling force for adolescent female promiscuity to seek survival with their bodies, and at the same time using the same reason to account for late marriages of young adult males who see the alternate route of illegal sex relationship as a way out of the crisis, and the lack of awareness on the part of the youths or teenagers on sex related issues.[248]

Adolescents could not really argue their position on this point beyond their understanding of what causes sexual promiscuity amongst youths-which they attributed much to the socio-economic situation of the country. Their position supports most of the arguments above.

Feminist, orthodox health experts and other antagonists of female circumcision argue that tradition has not been able to establish concrete relationship between uncut clitoris and promiscuity; and that proponents of female circumcision have their ideas borne out of the earlier lack of scientific knowledge and cultural taboos and restrictions on sex talks that impeded discussions on sexual pleasures arising from the clitoris in the woman in traditional societies. But that, with the gradual waning of such cultural hindrances and scientific knowledge, things are beginning to change. It is in their views that, there is the need for women to enjoy sex like men and that the idea of equating female circumcision with that of male has been condemned by both feminist and scientific researches. They argue that, since the penis itself is not excised or any portion but the foreskin, and sexual pleasure is maintained as well as fertility and general physical well-being, the two practices are incomparable.[249]

(3). Female circumcision is a male dictated and controlled aspect of the culture of the practicing areas.

Discourse

In discussing this stated hypothesis, the researcher asked female respondents, if they would circumcise their female children? Their responses ranged from 'if my husband insist, I would do it to protect our relationship; if it is going to affect our marriage I will have no choice; since men are difficult to find I will not like to

---

[247] Nahid Toubia 1993, Pp. 19.

[248] Ogor Alubo 2000, Pp. 6.

[249] Sanderson L. Passmore 1981, Pp. 17.

lose mine on account of insistence etc.' It is also expressed in an extreme form amongst the Urhobo and Okpe women that, upon penetrating un-excised woman, the man could be killed by secretion of a poison from the clitoris at the moment of contact with the penis. These sort of responses have been revealed in previous studies, that "common criticisms of the international move to ban female circumcision originate mostly from African women both those working to protect the cultural rite of passage and those forming and leading groups in their homelands to ban the practices. African women opposed to female circumcision contend that the issue is an internal one, connected to generations of power imbalances in relations between sexes and the social status of most women."[250]

Even older adult females connect their reasons to such issues like, 'uncircumcised woman finds it difficult to get married to a man; commands less respect before men and women folk alike among others.' This same cultural belief is evident in the practice among the Kenya ethnic groups of Maasai, and Meru.[251] While younger and older adult males who believe in the practice see it as a means of checking adultery, curbing sexual promiscuity and excessive sexual urges in order to protect or secure the masculine sexual dominance over the woman.

It should be noted, that female circumcision has been legitimised and sustained amongst the Okpe, and Urhobo speaking ethnic groups on the basis of the patriarchal nature of their societies. The socio-cultural, economic and political structures of these ethnic groups are controlled by, men. The gender phenomenon favours the male children in these two ethnic groups. More so, it is the same set of individuals that possess the cultural authority and dictate what constitute an establish culture and tradition of female sexuality. However, the few women who have attained social-political status in these ethnic communities must have among other conditions undergone female circumcision. This situation enhances in its intricate form the practice of female circumcision and other reproductive health issues that affect the girl child.[252]

Since traditional and cultural societies of Urhobo, Okpe, Isoko and Bini people are mainly male dominated and all norms, values, folklores, folktales are dictates from this 'gender favoured class' (men), and very few women in such positions the practice and continuation of female circumcision have always been vehemently defended by this category of individual. This is consistent with the position of feminist scholars, who argue that, the society is patriarchal in its organization, in that male dominance is institutionalised throughout the system, so much that the pursuit of universal perspectives on knowledge and issues affecting women are enveloped by belief systems and ways of functioning that

---

[250] Seble Dawit and Salem Mekuria 1993, Pp. 23.
[251] Jane N. Chege, et al. 2001, Pp. 10-12.
[252] Fikree F. Fariyal, et al. 2001, Pp. 134.

are fashioned by coalition of men and few women in positions of power to determine and control the fate of women in their own affairs.[253]

The older generation Urhobo, Okpe, Bini and Isoko women pride themselves in this virtue and honour of circumcision. They see it as their own status symbol of power, and help in supporting the male position for the continuation of the practice.

Those who argue against the practice, advocate a restructuring of the social - cultural framework of these ethnic groups. Even efforts by western feminists, non-governmental organizations, and 'official' institutions to protect women's human rights treat female circumcision in vacuum, advocating the disappearance of the practice without confronting the fundamental social framework that contains the ritual.[254]

(4). That there is a relationship between female circumcision and survival of the child during birth

Discourse

The Urhobo speaking people especially hold the firm cultural belief that it is impossible for an uncircumcised female to give birth to a life baby because when her uncut clitoris touches the forehead of the child during birth, the child will die. Thus, the uncut clitoris is believed to obstruct the birth passage of the child and makes delivery difficult. Though, the other ethnic groups like Okpe, Isoko and Bini speaking people use to hold a similar cultural belief to sustain the practice, I observed during my interviews that many of the proponents of this practice in these ethnic groups are beginning to undermine that aspect of traditional argument. Though, this same belief is held by practicing ethnic groups in Kenya, most documented scientific researches have contradicted this cultural belief system by arguing that, female genital mutilation can result in obstetrical complications for the mother and the fetus/baby e.g. delayed second stage labour, peri-natal tearing, vesico vagina fistula and low birth weight babies.[255] There were even situations where many uncircumcised women from circumcision practicing communities and ethnic groups like Jesse (a small Urhobo community in Ethiope-East) have been reported to have had children without circumcising. This was confirmed by an Urhobo indigenous orthodox female health expert and one of my case study- an adolescent female who hails from an Urhobo community and family, where the practice of female circumcision is deeply entrenched, but herself uncircumcised and currently nursing a child of about a year and half.

The idea is that tradition and cultural argument for legitimising the practice are not concrete as they adopt horror trips as strategies to sustain the practice in

---

[253] Rich, 1993, Pp. 1123.
[254] Nina B. Huntemann 1995, Pp. 36.
[255] B. Calder, et al. 1993, Pp. 712-716.

order to integrate others to the old belief system. One of the younger adults female, Miss Imen opined, that:

> '...One would have thought that the uncircumcised females do not give birth at all until they were circumcised. This inconsistency in the traditional belief about female circumcision is questionable...'

Similar views were held by orthodox health experts and younger adults, that even among the Urhobo, Okpe, Bini, Ika and other female circumcision practicing communities, children die during childbirth, and this was often as a result of mishandling of the entire birth process by either orthodox or unorthodox health expert providers, which maybe due to poor facilities and lack of adequate knowledge and training.[256] Early documented researches also point out that, circumcised mothers are more likely to die from childbirth due to a re-tear of the vagina and resultant excessive bleeding or haemorrhage.[257]

Thus the fear of social criticisms and the stigmatisation of uncircumcised females are some of the reasons for evoking such ideas to horrify the females for the purpose of social integration in the society.

11.2.b. Medical Hypotheses on Female Circumcision

(5). That circumcised females are easily prone to HIV/AIDS infections.

Discourse

Orthodox health experts claimed a medical possibility for the spread of the HIV/AIDS through contact of the circumcised female who suffers a re-tear of the vagina during sexual intercourse with an infected man, and the use of infected instrument to circumcise multiple individuals. The re-tear of the vagina after circumcision, is a very high possibility on two conditions, first during childbirth and second, during sexual intercourse with a man that is infected and at the same time has very large penis. Documented studies have corroborated the possibilities anticipated by the orthodox health experts. Research studies carried out on 7, 350 young girls less than 16 years old in Dar -Es- Salem showed that female circumcision might play a role in the transmission of HIV; as it revealed that 97 percent of the time the same un-sterilized equipment could be used for the circumcision on 15 – 20 girls. The study revealed further that the same equipment facilitated HIV/AIDS/STD transmission.[258] Another study conducted in Nairobi revealed that, female circumcision predisposes women to HIV infection in many ways e.g. increase need for blood transfusions due to hemorrhage either when the procedure is performed, at childbirth, or as a result of vagina tearing during de-infibulation and intercourse, and the use of the same un-sterilized instruments for other initiates.[259]

---

[256] Valentine Otoide, et al. 2001, Pp. 81.

[257] C. Oyugi 1998, Pp. 1011.

[258] I. B. Mutenbi and M. K. Nwesiga 1998, Pp. 436.

[259] C. Oyugi, 1998, Pp. 1011-1012.

The research study results above, is a potent reality in the Nigerian society particularly, in the Northern part of the country where child marriages and female circumcision is a known dominant practice aided by culture, religion and tradition. More so, as the awareness level of the HIV/AIDS virus is still very low, and yet the level of adolescent sexual activities is very high, and the equipment for handling circumcision are the same for multiple individuals under cultural interpretation of rituals, and cannot be reliably said to be infection free. All of these pose great dangers to the health of the adolescent female in particular and the populace in general.

Though there are controversies at socio-medical, health and reproductive experts level on the predominance of the spread of HIV/AIDS in non-practicing female circumcision regions of Africa, such as eastern Zaire, Rwanda, Burundi, western Uganda, north-western Tanzania, and northern Zambia.[260] Health experts argue that it is not enough to play down the outright consequences of the continuity of the practice of female circumcision with the reality that HIV/AIDS is a potential source for the ease of transmission of the virus[261] especially, among the Urhobo, Okpe and Isoko practising ethnic groups where group circumcision by traditional midwives is still a cherished custom with more or less un-sterilized equipment.

(6). That female circumcision is carried out more by traditional midwives and native doctors.

Discourse

Both orthodox and unorthodox health experts accuse each other for the perpetuation of the dangerous and complicated form of female circumcision. To establish a fact on this, the researcher asked the question to all category of participants especially circumcised females where and who circumcised them?

The answers were varied as the number of participants. Even adolescent and adult male participants were equally asked where their sisters (if any), wives (if any) or daughters (if any) respectively, were circumcised and by whom? I recorded that both the orthodox and unorthodox health experts shared proportionately in the mention as part of the process of providing circumcision services.

Even in this circumstance, the orthodox health experts accused the trado-medical practitioners for perpetuating the dangerous and complicated form of female circumcision.

Two of the female traditional midwives accepted to have engaged in the act of female circumcision as part of their services to clients. One claimed to have quitted from the practice for personal health reasons (weak sight) while the other still does it as a veritable source of her income. Evidence abound in many studies that most female circumcisions are carried out by traditional midwives in Eritrea,

---

[260] G. Pieters 1972, Pp 173 / J. A. Verzin 1975, Pp. 163.
[261] Daniel B. Hrdy 1987, Pp. 1109.

Cote d' Ivoire, Mali, Kenya and Nigeria; and tools such as razor baldes, knives, sharp stones, broken bottles, scissors, un-sterilized without anaesthesia are used.[262]

The two male trado-medical expert expressed confidence in the act of female circumcision carried out by traditional midwives. Chief Oko stated that twenty-two of his female children went through the act in the hands of traditional midwives without any complications. The other (Chief Jon) claimed same, for his daughters and younger wives.

Three of the orthodox health experts accepted that some of their colleagues are implicated in the act of female circumcision due to pressures from parents of victims and the financial benefits, even with their knowledge of the health implications. In a country, like Egypt where the practice of female circumcision is supported with Islamic religious interpretation, orthodox health providers like doctors, midwives and nurses engage in the circumcision of females, and it is believed that this trend might reduce the pains, risks and complications that is associated with it.[263] They condemned those involved in very strong terms as breaching the medical ethics. Feminist writers, who argues in a critique of international attempts to regulate female circumcision in practicing communities warns that, "approaching clitoridectomy as a health issue raises concern. If the practice could be done without negative health consequences, international law might actually become complicit in the practice, obligating states to ensure that it is performed under better health conditions."[264]

What is not in contention in practicing communities is that both orthodox and unorthodox health experts (mostly women) are today involved in providing the services of female circumcision. The only contentious fact is that of proportion which approximates more in number of traditional midwives as the perpetrators of dangerous forms of circumcision with the use of crude methods.[265]

However, educational level of parents influences decision of where, and how parents want the act to be done on their child. Also, studies have shown that most of those engaged in the practice – traditionalist, orthodox health experts, and victims do it for the economic gains and benefits derived, as it serves one major source of income for traditional midwives while it helped to augment the incomes of orthodox health providers involved in the act, and victims and their families received gifts in terms of food, materials and even monies.[266]

---

[262] Fran P. Hosken 1993, Pp. 3.
[263] MYWO and PATH 1991, Pp. 18.
[264] Karen Engle 1992, Pp. 1515.
[265] Fran P. Hosken 1989, Pp. 3-12.
[266] S. Robinson 2001, Pp. 3.

11.2.c. Legislative Hypotheses on Female Circumcision

(7). Adolescent females are subjected to the act of circumcision against their consent.

Discourse

To establish the validity of the above hypothesis, adolescent females were asked questions such as; at what age were you circumcised; who was instrumental to your circumcision; would you have circumcised if given the choice?

In answer to these questions, nine out of twelve adolescent females who had circumcised gave varied age range from under to over age depending on the ethnic group and the community from which they hailed from. They also mentioned those instrumental for their circumcision; and the reasons given for their circumcision were listed in the following order,

- Parental influence and coercion
- Conditions given by tradition for marriage
- Mother-in-law threats to their daughter -in-laws, son-in-laws, and granddaughters (grand parents influence)

Previous studies stated that, "most girls undergo female circumcision when they are very young especially between the ages of 7 and 10 years old."[267] Further studies have shown that female circumcision seem to be occurring at early ages in several countries because parents want to reduce the trauma on their children and to avoid government interference where laws exist against the practice and also, to avoid or prevent the resistance of children when they grow old enough to form their own opinion.[268] Some women are coerced to undergo female circumcision during early adulthood when marrying into a community that practices female circumcision or just before or after birth of a first child, like in some part of Mali and among the Urhobo and Ibo speaking ethnic groups in Delta and Eastern parts of Nigeria respectively.

Circumcised female adolescents reacted in consensus that given the choice they would not have circumcised. They call for females to be allowed to attain certain ages when they are capable of deciding if they wanted the act performed on them or not, if the practice is to be allowed to continue. Studies showed that the U.S. government reacted to the plights of adolescent females by passing a law in 1997 criminalizing female circumcision performed on a person who has not reached the age of 18 years but the law does not address women who are older than 18 years. However, it is believed that at age 18 one was old enough to make personal and reasonable choices and decisions. Even, most developed countries such as Canada, Sweden, England, Australia, have made statutes prohibiting female circumcision and re-infibulation after delivery.[269]

---

[267] Demographic Health Survey (DHS) 1995, Pp. 175.

[268] Fran P. Hosken 1993, Pp. 35.

[269] Margaret Brady 1999, Pp. 715.

Even young adolescent females whose culture abhors female circumcision accepted during discussion session that if "not circumcising their daughters would result in a threat to marital stability or threaten the possibility of getting married or serves as a condition for getting married, they would have no choice in their words 'but to do it' to their daughters, only if they had tried to convince their boy friends or husband and it failed". Younger unmarried adult females bracket shared similar sentiments with the above position. What is reinforced is the same old prejudice about the myth of male superiority.[270] This male superiority is predominant especially among the Urhobo, Okpe, Bini, and Isoko ethnic groups in Nigeria

Older adult females insist on the circumcision of their granddaughters if their parents failed to do it. They believe that it does not only help to curb promiscuity of the female but to increase the marriage prospect of the girl and consequently the bride wealth to the family of the girl. In fact, studies on Egypt women show that most women who have undergone the procedure are strongly in favour of the female circumcision for their daughters and granddaughters.[271]

Older adult males were resolute in their stance that their daughters and wives must undergo the process without questioning, and they frowned at anti-female circumcision advocates for not understanding the social framework and context in which they are fighting. They understand the campaign as a challenge to cultural sovereignty and an interference of westerners on indigenous culture.[272]

Thus the idea that female circumcision still plays an active role in the determination of marriage, the social pressure and stigma attached to uncircumcised females, and the insistence of mother-in-laws to carry out the act on their granddaughters by issuing all forms of threats, and the influences of gender favour of the male child in this respect, as well as the lack of choice of the female child in the determination of whether the act be performed on her or not, indicates that female children are circumcised against their consents and in most cases by coercion. However, Female circumcision would have to be abolished if the opinion of young people from Urhobo, Isoko, Okpe, Bini, and Ika are considered against their uniform opposition to the practice in their various ethnic groups.

(8). Adolescents advocate a legislative policy to ban the practice of female circumcision.

Discourse

This hypothesis was discussed analytically with the exclusive opinions of the adolescents. To understand their perspective on a legislation to ban or continue the practice of female circumcision; adolescents (male and females) were asked

---

[270] DHS 1989-1990, Pp. 124.
[271] DHS 1995, Pp. 173.
[272] Seble Dawit and Salem Mekuria 1993, Pp. 27.

the following questions; would you like female circumcision to continue or not? How do you think female circumcision could be discouraged? What other contributions would you like to make towards the current debate on discouraging or encouraging female circumcision?

Their answers were disproportionate in favour of more adolescents calling for legislation to ban outright the practice of female circumcision. Sixteen out of seventeen adolescent participants (male and female) were unanimous in advocating for an effective legislation to ban the practice because of the associated health hazard. This constitutes about 94.1 percent of the total adolescent respondents. While one adolescent male took a different stance by favouring the continuation of the practice for what he termed the numerous benefits. This number constitutes about 5.9 percents.

The position of adolescents advocating for a ban on the practice of female circumcision is overwhelming and this underscores the argument of orthodox health experts on the medical concerns of what they termed a 'dangerous traditional practice.' This lays a significant basis for a comprehensive strategy for educating both practicing and non-practicing female circumcision communities to understand the need for a change in attitude. Most research studies have chronicled the health dangers associated with the practice. Human right groups and concerned organizations have chronicled the abuse of the female body through circumcision as spelt out in the following; in the Universal Declaration of Human Rights (1948), United Nations Convention on the Rights of the Child (1959), the African Charter on Rights and Welfare of the Child (1990), the United Nations Convention on the Elimination of All Forms of Discriminations against Women (1992), the United Nations Declaration on Violence Against Women (1993); the World Conference on Human Rights, Declarations and Programme of Action, Vienna (1993) etc. and have also recommended a change in attitude through enlightenment and education of practicing communities. Coupled with these, many studies argue, for effective legislations to be promulgated in areas yet to have one to ensure a positive campaign against the practice, and make effective implementations of the laws already existing where the practice has been ban,[273] otherwise, the practicing ethnic groups would resort to clandestine and crude methods which might be more dangerous in to the victims and complicate their health.

---

[273] Nahid Toubia 1993, Pp. 44 / MFAD, 1995, Pp. 17.

11.3. Evaluation of the General assumptions of Reproductive Health

This study examined the five stated general assumptions on adolescent reproductive health in Nigeria.

(a) Education and Adolescent reproductive Health

Though young people are aware of certain reproductive health information like abortion and female circumcision in Nigeria. What they know is inadequate and from informal sources. This lack of adequate education on reproductive health information has slowed the pace of change with little or no significant forward movement, reflecting the controversies that remain around sexuality and reproductive health and rights. The difficulty of discussing adolescent sexual and reproductive health and the challenges of protecting young peoples right while respecting parental responsibilities are critical factors that has contributed to this slow pace of improvement in adolescent reproductive health. While studies still continue to show that adolescent who receive sexual and reproductive health education and information and services are more likely to delay sexual activity, have fewer sexual partners, are less likely to engage in risky sexual behaviour, and are less likely to have unplanned pregnancies or contract STDs (Family Care International 2001), the situation of adolescent reproductive health in Nigeria is shrouded in cultural myths and taboos. This contradicts the International Conference on Population and Development (ICPD) programme of Action paragraph 7.41 which states "…information and services should be made available to adolescents to help them understand their sexuality and protect themselves from unwanted pregnancies, sexually transmitted diseases and subsequent risk of infertility. This should be combined with the education of young men to respect women's self-determination and to share responsibility with women in matters of sexuality and reproduction."

This situation poses future challenges to the Nigerian health institutions, since any effort to address adolescent reproductive health must acknowledge the realities of adolescent sexuality and young peoples specific health needs. Programmes that involve adolescents in design and delivery of education and care, as well as built systems of support among teachers, parents and communities must be encouraged. Education on reproductive health must overcome a considerable range of challenges by recognising the following,

- that adolescent sexuality and needs for reproductive health services are still sensitive issues among policy makers, parents, community leaders and teachers
- that cultures and religious fundamentalism (Christianity and Islam) discouraging or preventing adolescents from receiving sexuality education and sexual reproductive health services should be enlightened and educated, and
- health workers should be educated to provide services to adolescents and young peoples even when such cultural restriction exists.

All these would be possible if only education in its elaborate form is 'massified.' That is education should be made compulsory and possibly free at the primary and secondary school levels for all irrespective of gender, and an incorporated curriculum on reproductive health in the syllabus at those levels. The situation in Nigeria where education at these levels is still not reachable to the large number of people because of the high cost, is a major handicap to this sensitive bracket of society- the adolescents who are vulnerable victims of sexual and reproductive health problems. Thus whether adolescents have the reproductive health education and services that they need, and the health care and economic opportunity to lead fulfilling lives in Nigeria, depends on the action of the government in educating the great mass of people which begin at the very rudimentary level of primary and secondary institutions, with emphasis on sexuality and reproductive health issues.

(b) Parental Factor and Adolescent reproductive Health

Parents are very important in the socialization or upbringing of the child. Unfortunately, the viewpoint of parents on adolescent reproductive health and sexual development has been that of evasion. For instance, a greater proportion of parents in Nigeria do not favour the use of contraceptives by sexually active adolescents because according to them contraception kills. Also, most do not usually discuss sexual matters with their adolescent girls.[274] Contradictorily, the same majority of parents would want a sex education program in schools in order to prevent unwanted pregnancies, and other harmful reproductive health problems.[275]

In Nigeria, despite some form of eroding traditional values especially, in the urban centres, parents still have a tremendous influence over their children. Therefore, meeting the reproductive health needs of adolescents mostly rest on their shoulders at the beginning. Most parents or guardians do not or avoid discussions of sexual matters with their daughters or wards as a result of shyness, ignorance on sexual matters or societal norms that do not encourage open-mother-with daughter discussion on sexual issues. Much more than cultural and societal norm restrictions, is the fact that most parents are embarrassed to discuss such issues with their daughters or wards.

Taking into considerations the delay or deliberate avoidance on the part of government to implement the series of international resolutions on the reproductive health rights of the adolescent, the opinion and attitude of parents specifically, towards sexual and reproductive health matters with their daughters could play a significant role in reducing the numerous problems that result from reproductive and sexual health hazards like unwanted pregnancies, illegal abortions, use of ineffective contraceptives, contraction of infectious diseases like STDs, AIDS/HIV, female genital mutilation etc. Parental influence and

[274] L. A. Briggs 1998, Pp. 262.
[275] Ibid 1998, Pp. 265.

cooperation would also help in the implementation of meaningful family planning programmes directed towards adolescents and initiated from the primary agent or basis of socialization-the family, rather than expose the adolescent to other indirect and dangerous sources of procuring information.

Parents with negative notions on sexual and reproductive health issues in Nigeria, need to be aware of the importance of reproductive health education if there are to play a vital role in socializing their wards to prevent emerging future reproductive health problems. They should realise that learning about sexuality is a life long process and a fundamental part of every person's socialization.[276]

(c) Community and Religious Leaders and Adolescent Reproductive Health
Most health policy thrust in Nigeria have consistently omitted the incorporation and opinions of traditional, community and religious leaders in the mobilization process for campaigns against obnoxious and harmful traditional reproductive health practices that affect the adolescent in general and the females in particular. Attempt to improve adolescent reproductive health should ensure a strong consensus of all shed of opinion particularly, with these groups of leaders who still enjoys the respect and support of the people in all moral issues, especially, in sexual and reproductive health matters. Thus, these individual wield significant influence in the 'change process' of society. To omit this group of individuals who have led successful campaigns in other sub-Saharan African countries like Sierra-Leone, Senegal, Mali and countries like Kenya against harmful female circumcision practices undermines the notion of active and responsive participation of all in the change process. This has been one of the banes in the successful campaign against harmful traditional health practices like female circumcision, abortion and contraceptives usage among adolescents in general and the girl child in particular, among many Nigeria ethnic groups like Igbo, Urhobo, Bini, Isoko, Yoruba and Hausa to mention but a few.

Consequently, recognition and incorporation of these groups of individuals in enlightenment and awareness programmes in Nigeria, where over 48 per cent of the people are Christians and about 50 per cents are Islamic adherents, and both combine in their various capacities traditional worships, such efforts at the recognition of their leaders as target in the enlightenment and educational awareness programme has the ability to effectively mobilise the masses and disseminate appropriate information on contraceptive usage (e.g. condoms); and abrogation of harmful traditional reproductive health practices like female circumcision in practicing communities. This is because the religious institutions remain the cornerstone of many Nigerian communities and most community leaders even seek leadership from the churches in these days.

(d) Improved Socio-Economic Status of Women and Reproductive Health
The low status of women in most of the ethnic groups in Nigeria- especially among the Urhobo, Bini, Igbo, Yoruba, and Hausa speaking people continues to

---

[276] G. H. Allan, et al. 1998, Pp. 3.

decline in spite of efforts by women groups and non-governmental organizations campaign for improvement in their status. This situation contradicts the Article 1, of the United Nations, Convention on the Elimination of All Forms of Discrimination against Women (The Women's Convention) that was adopted by the United Nations General Assembly in 1979. The Convention defines discrimination against women as "...any distinction, exclusion, or restriction made on the basis of sex which has the effect or purpose of impairing or nullifying the recognition, enjoyment or exercise by women, irrespective of their marital status, on a basis of equality of men and women of human rights and fundamental freedoms in political, economic, social, cultural, civil or any other field."

Throughout their life cycle, the Nigerian woman daily existence and long term aspirations are restricted by discriminatory attitudes, unjust social and economic structures, and a lack of resources that prevent their full and equal participation in the community. This contradiction in article 1, continually affect the social and economic independence of the Nigerian woman. This makes them to be dependent on men even on issues that affect them, particularly in the area of reproductive health. Decision that affect their bodies are thus at the privy of gender bias, culture and societal dictates.

An obligation of state parties to revert the trend of women status for the better by taking appropriate measures to eliminate the discrimination against women by improving their socio-economic status through improvement in their education, access and equal opportunities to better jobs, equal opportunities to political positions etc. can empower women and help them to be active participants in taking control of matters that affect their sexual and reproductive health rights. Thus the power relations that impede women's attainment of a healthy and fulfilling life operate at many levels of society, from the most personal to the highly public. Consequently, improving the status of women would enhance their decision-making capacity at all levels and in all aspects of life, especially in the area of sexuality and reproduction.

(e) Government Implementation of Reproductive Health Policies
One critical factor that affects adolescent female reproductive health in Nigeria is the inactive and irresponsive attitude of the national government to the commitment of the series of international resolution that she was a party. A chronicle of some of the international resolutions include the United nations, Convention on the Elimination of All Forms of Discrimination against the Women, adopted in 1979; The International Conference on Population and Development (ICPD) in 1994 Programme of Action, Paragraph 7.41 containing "information and services to be made available to adolescents, to help them understand their sexuality and protect themselves from unwanted pregnancies, sexually transmitted diseases, and subsequent risk of infertility..."; The 1995 Fourth World Conference on Women in Beijing; The Women Convention on Human Rights, otherwise known as the Vienna Declaration and Program of

Action which for the first time recognised that women have right to 'the highest standard of physical and mental health throughout their life span', and on the basis of equality between women and men, 'a right to accessible and adequate health care and the widest range of family planning services...' etc. Even the Nigerian Constitution guaranteed enforceable equal rights in these respects. Though, she has not registered any reservations to these international conventions and resolutions it was clear that the government was not complying with the provisions. Unfortunately, it is a country deeply steeped in traditions.

However, the conferences together have provided firm basis for establishing women's right to sexual and reproductive health. Government irresponsiveness to these resolutions is a significant factor that has serious implications on important institutions and non-governmental organizations (NGOs) that are genuinely committed to the course of elimination of all forms of discriminations on reproductive and sexual health issues that affect the adolescent female in particular. Consequently, if the Nigerian government take all appropriate measures to be committed religiously to all resolutions in this respect to eliminate discrimination against adolescent females in particular in the field of reproductive health care by ensuring a basis of equality of men and women, access to health services, there would be a tremendous improvement in the sexual and reproductive health of adolescents in general and the female in particular.

12.0. Chapter twelve
Discussions, Recommendations and Conclusion
12.1. Discussion
The greatest advantage of this research is the use of the qualitative techniques of data collection to understand the socio-cultural, political and economic environment of the research areas on adolescent reproductive health issues. More so, this enabled the adolescent respondents to bare their minds on the issues raised along with the views of adults, orthodox and unorthodox health experts, legal practitioners, legislators, women and human rights activists.

Most ethnic communities in Nigeria like the Urhobo and Okpe are still somewhat traditional in their structure. It was observed during the focus group discussions, personal interviews, and case studies sessions that most issues relating to reproductive health in terms of sexual behaviour, abortion, female circumcision are still regarded as traditional and religious taboos and there are restrictions in discussions on such by adolescents females and males or women in the society. It is the prerogative of the man who is regarded as the head of the family to control or direct discussions on such issues. This makes it very difficult for women to freely participate in the discussions of issues that concern them. Experience has shown that women are quite freer to speak on issues of sexuality when no man is around. This position agrees with previous researches on reproductive health and women fertility that, there is no significant association between contraceptives use and women's discussion with their husband about family size and family planning, which have been found to be important for predicting fertility change.[277] In effect, patriarchal and patrilocal family structure still appears to have strong influence on reproductive health decision- making.

Another exceptional issue is the finding of the conflicting perspectives of respondents relating to women's autonomy. The lack of the autonomy on the part of the Urhobo, Okpe or Bini woman, result in their lower socio-economic status which makes them to be unable to have direct influence on their participation in institutions- political, economic, social or health to make valuable decisions that concern their bodies- particularly, in the area of reproductive health matters like abortion and female circumcision. Some socio-economic obstacles hindering women's participation in the decision on reproductive health matters in these ethnic communities include,

- Poverty and unemployment
- Lack of adequate financial resources
- Illiteracy, semi illiteracy and choice of profession
- The dual burden of domestic task and professional obligation
- Laws and government policies that are gender sensitive.

Although, the importance of women's biological and social roles are clear their inputs in all sectors of life in Nigeria often goes unrecognised. For instance in the

---

[277] Fikree F. Fariyal, et al. 2001, Pp. 134-135.

third year of Nigeria fourth democratic republic, the composition of the National Assembly show that in the senate, only 3 out of the 109 members are women and 12 out of 360 are members of the lower house (house of representative); and among the 40 ministers in the federal executive, there are 4 substantive female ministers, 3 ministers of state, 4 female advisers/presidential assistants. At the state level, there are 15 women in all the 36 state houses of assembly out of a grand total of 978 members (one of them a deputy speaker of the house), and only one of them is a deputy governor of a state. In all the 774 local government, there are only 3 female chairpersons (called chairmen), out of a total of 8,657 local councillors, 143 are women.[278] As few as they are in number considering that women constitutes about half of the Nigerian population, and are just as educated as the men, they are often in conflict when it came to taking a consensus position on decisions affecting their reproductive health. The strength of this study is to specify these figures as revealed, on factors that affect population policies and the reproductive health of females in Nigeria particularly with respect to the debate on liberalization or legalization of abortion and legislation against female circumcision. The crucial issue is, not that there is a lack of attention to the issue of poverty, reproductive health matters and other problems that affects women, but rather the imminent conflict that arises among the few privileged women, the male folks and the non-commitment in most cases to addressing these problems by legislative authorities.

Some general Socio-cultural obstacle which affect enactments of laws, on female reproductive health, in Nigeria include,

- Culture used as religion- especially, the spread of fundamental Islam in the form of Sharia; and spread of fundamental Christianity in the Northern and Southern states of Nigeria respectively, predetermined social roles assigned to women, which results in women lack of confidence in themselves and their subordinate status
- The lack of respectability in presenting or portraying the image of the woman in public
- The segregated roles for the sexes as enforced by traditional cultural values, which places the men as superior to the female and,

The socio-cultural values militate against the advancement, progress and participation of females on matters that affect them. This socio-cultural handicap also manifested during the focus group discussions with adolescent males and females. For instance in most responses, the males saw themselves in control of issues that concern sexual and reproductive health matters. Even the female respondents showed lack of confidence on matters that affected them particularly- like female circumcision and abortion. For instance, most of them agreed to cede their opinion of circumcising their female children to their husband if it would threaten or endangers their marital or friendly relationship.

---

[278] Stella Omu 2000, Pp. 16.

However, it was obvious during the discussion with respondents that adolescents generally who were from average socio-economic background and from urban schools were better informed on the issues of abortion and female circumcision than those from the lower socio-economic background and from interior or rural schools in the local government areas of study. This sharp divide could be attributed to the poor socio-economic environment that translates to lack of modern informational facilities and infra-structural facilities.

The modernity versus traditional divide was significant in the generational comparison of reproductive health issues of the female. On the issue of the continuous practice of female circumcision and the liberalization of female circumcision, older adults toed the position of culture and tradition to embellish their views while the youths (adolescents and younger adults) hinged their arguments on contemporary developments and the health implications of the practice.

The emphasis on 'marriage before sex' was a tool highlighted by adults. To them it did not matter what age the individual started having sex so long as they were married. Their nostalgic relapse to tradition to support their view, distinct them from the adolescent who indicate a social acceptance of premarital sex. Adults defined 'sexual responsibility' in terms of marriage and not age. Abortion to the older adults was out-rightly condemned as wrong and against tradition and the spilling of human blood. It was observed that these same adults always resorted to adopting the recommendation of education and enlightenment (which are effective tools of modernization) of adolescent on reproductive health matters in the event that the traditional explanation for the continuation of female circumcision and the perpetuation of illegal abortion amongst the adolescents failed, because of the grave health consequences. This drift in position conflicts with their concept of the mystification of sex related issues as taboos. Their call for the medicalization of the operational procedure of female circumcision rather than abrogate a 'valued cultural practice' is another revelation of their conflicting perspectives of modernization and tradition.

Both orthodox and unorthodox expert health providers agreed that illegal abortion and the dangerous processes of female circumcision could endanger the health of the girl child. But they both disagree on the approach to rectify the issues.

The issue of Polygamy was a predominant feature observed in the family structure of most Nigerian communities. The forty-four respondents in the varied category of data collection techniques were either directly or indirectly from a polygamous background. They were either from a polygamous parentage, or themselves polygamist by marriage or the women married to polygamous men or socialized in a polygamous environment. But while polygamy by the man is accepted by society as morally right, it is the reverse with the female. This has a major implication on the views of both males and female respondents. For instance, the adolescent male has no regrets in keeping multiple relationships for the purpose of just 'enjoying himself', while the same situation when applicable to the adolescent female is considered as immoral act even when done for both economic and emotional reasons. Thus, the greatest victims of polygamy are the females who suffer lower status as a result of this act by men. This is one reason women compromise their position or stance on reproductive health matters that affects them. They are prepared to suffer the emotional, economic and psychological stress and get used to their husband for fear of losing favour from him to the benefit of other women. The idea is that the man could always have another woman while it would be impossible for her to get same. The health implication of this is for the woman to expect an easy infection with sexually transmitted diseases like STD's and HIV/AIDS virus because of the promiscuity of the man.

Religious practices like Christianity and Islam impacted on the ideas of all the respondents. My notations during focus group discussions, personal interviews and case studies sessions with respondents revealed that those who oppose liberalization or legalization of abortion and legislation against female circumcision misconceive religion on the issues. They use religion to colour and support their argument on issues of reproductive health of the female. This has a serious implication in influencing government positions and policy makers in their formulation of health policies. With respect to female circumcision, it was observed that a woman's mother-in-law has very strong influence on couple reproductive decision- making. This is because of the existing patriarchal and patrilocal family structure existing in most Nigeria communities especially, amongst the Urhobo and Okpe peoples. Consequently, the old generation women in these areas kick hard against any policy that is proposed to outlaw female circumcision. Most of them have been brainwashed by their husbands and men to believe in the sanctity of the practice, and to see it as a symbol of women power, honour and pride, and that women cannot take a political position in the community unless they were excised, at which point some of them are subjected to an oath of secrecy. This aspect is crucial in the case of initiating change and identifying target interventions.

12.2. Recommendations

The factors that affect adolescent females reproductive health revolve around the biological, social, religion, economic, cultural and environmental and these must be aggressively addressed if significant improvement is to occur in their health and welfare. Despite efforts by governments to remain committed to the basic tenets of the Beijing Platform of Action (BPFA), the International Conference on Population and Development in Cairo, and all other international resolutions on women welfare, the fact remains that adolescent females health are still grossly underrepresented in policy decisions. This study recommends the following:

(a) Education and Enlightenment

The issue of adolescents female reproductive health with respect to the twin issues of legalization or liberalization of abortion and legislation against female circumcision can be attained with the improved greater education and enlightenment of women in particular, and the society in general. This would create awareness on the dangers of illegal abortion and the health hazard associated with female circumcision. Education would also improve and elevate the status of women and consequently, improve their reproductive health. Formal education and training of women is an important precondition for their development and gender -balanced representation on decision- making boards on health matters.

This form of education will also make the woman to be socially aware of traditionally assigned gender roles that tended to limit their choices in education and career. More so, it would help women themselves to initiate challenges to the patriarchal structures and beliefs and the ideological frameworks that perpetuates women's view of their seemingly natural subordinate position. The form of education should also take the following form,

- Expand the capacity of education systems and make them more flexible in meeting the learning and other needs of girls
- Make education more gender sensitive throughout with special attention to the nature of the school environment (particularly their safety and security), teaching and learning processes, and the education context
- Socialize both boys and girls in learning environments which are non violent and encourage mutual respect, dignity and equality
- Include sex education in the academic curricula at the secondary school levels.

Education and awareness campaigns should target the rural populace where over 75 percent of the female population as well as traditional, community and opinion leaders reside. In this context, most of the staunch antagonists to reformist policies on harmful traditional and cultural practices like female circumcision would be effectively targeted.

More so, all forms of awareness and enlightenment campaigns should emphasize on the dangers associated with female reproductive health matters like illegal abortion, female circumcision, unwanted pregnancies, sex behaviour etc. rather than targeting the culture or tradition of female circumcision or the sanctity of life, which often provoke the people as an attack on their culture and tradition.

Traditional midwives who are mostly implicated for the perpetuation of the surgical operation of female circumcision should be targeted and incorporated into awareness and enlightenment campaign programs. Efforts should be made to create alternative jobs or occupations for them in other sectors of the economy like providing them with financial supports to embark on petty trading in order to divert their attention from engaging in the hazardous female reproductive health practices like female circumcision and the perpetuation of dangerous and illegal abortion, which they see as a means of earning income rather than the conviction of the usefulness of the practice.

Television remains an important medium to educate and communicate with the adolescents, while radios and newspapers are more attractive appeals to villagers and literate adults respectively. The focus of the campaign should be on the dangers of illegal abortion, female circumcision and other harmful traditional reproductive health practices that affect the girl child. The mode of language should be the adoption of the 'Pidgin English' (i.e. a form of corrupted English Language) because it is widely spoken by over 97percent of the entire Nigerian populace. Thus its wide outreach, acceptance and understanding would serve as an added advantage by saving costs of translation of messages to the more than 350 existing ethnic languages in Nigeria. Though at the college levels, the English language should be used as effective complement to the 'pidgin English' for sex education lectures because of the academic environment. The use of town criers in villages, magazines publications, theatres, dramas, film shows, arts works and photographs should be implored to display the dangers of the female circumcision and illegal abortion as well.

(b) Knowledge, Attitude and Practice of reproductive health

From my observation adolescent males and men generally were more likely than women to be aware of reproductive health matters. This is likely because of cultural and religious reasons in most of the ethnic groups particularly, among the Urhobo, Okpe and Bini that make women shy, timid and ashamed to open up their views on issues of sexuality. For instance, when they were asked about means of preventing pregnancies, issues on abortion and disease prevention, they had more knowledge on the use of condoms and pills, although there were not convinced on its application and efficacy. They (males) could tell where to procure abortion and contraceptives illegally for their girl friends unlike their female counterparts. Due to this significant observation, it is recommended that adolescent females be specifically targeted during enlightenment and educational campaigns on reproductive health issue and be allowed to have unrestricted access to the procurement of contraceptives as preventive techniques. The males should be encouraged to adopt contraceptive usage particularly the condom.

The majority of adolescents (males and females) and young adult males and females are opposed to female circumcision and agree that the practice be discontinued. These views would help to consolidate public opinion against female circumcision and to contribute to the legislative initiatives against the practice.

(c) Religious Misconceptions

This study recommends that policy makers in Nigeria should attempt to clarify religious misconceptions about female circumcision and the issue of illegal and unwanted pregnancies vis-à-vis other harmful female reproductive health practices by seeking the active collaboration and support of religious leaders, which has been done in Muslim countries such as Egypt, Indonesia, Senegal,

Turkey, Tunisia and Iran. In addition, the study recommends that researchers should be encouraged to conduct qualitative studies to explore the influence of religious beliefs on attitudes about female circumcision and illegal abortion, particularly amongst local Christian clerics, Islamic and other religious leaders. This is because of the severe connection between the law and religious institutions in Nigeria, and the influence, support and respects that the churches and Islamic leaders enjoy from the people. For instance, the use of the Sharia in the Northern part of Nigeria to sustain the argument for the practice of female circumcision and the use of the Christian religion in the Southern part of Nigeria to argue against any form of legislation against female circumcision or the liberalization of abortion should be thoroughly and religiously re-examined.

(d) The Law and Practice on Health Issues

There is a discrepancy between the law and practice or its application on issues of female reproductive health in Nigeria. Effort should be made by the government to implement effective laws that criminalize certain hazardous reproductive health practices that affect the woman. For instance, even when abortion is considered illegal by the law, there are clear evidences that it was still perpetuated secretly in private and public health institutions as well as traditional herbal homes by medical doctors, nurses, native doctors and traditional midwives. It is this secrecy in its perpetuation that account for unreported and unrecorded large number of teenage maternal deaths resulting from illegal and criminal abortion. This is one of the reason, advocates are calling for the liberalization of the law or legalization of it so that the process could be regulated openly to reduce the catastrophic number of deaths that results.

It is on records that female circumcision has been outlawed in only 3 states of the 36 states that make up the Nigerian federation namely, Edo, Delta and Ogun. Despite the existing legislations in place there are no effective means of monitoring the efficacy of the application of the sanctions prescribed by the law. It is important to mention, that the approved sanctions for culprits ranged from 2 to 3 years imprisonment or an option of fine of between #2,000 and #3,000 Naira. This is considered relatively minimal a punishment to make the law effective. Other loopholes in the law show that since the practice has not been outlawed in other part of the country, people still take their daughters from these areas where the laws are now in place to other states where the law is yet to apply to carry out the process of circumcision on their daughters. This is why it is recommended that a more national concern and outlook must be canvassed for a national law to be put in place to eradicate this practice that has been known to have a lot of dangerous health consequences on the girl child, and the law would be binding on all states of the federation. It is important that the act of female circumcision be criminalized nationally before the issue of effective implementation could be explored in detail.

The code of conducts of doctors should be reviewed to make them more effective health providers. This would help them to first take urgent medical decisions to save the life of a woman brought with complications of illegal abortion rather than emphasize on the detail inquiry of the source of the administration of the illegal abortion before treatment was administered because of the law. In the case of female circumcision, doctors should help in the enlightenment of parents, practising communities and other individuals who are still interested to seek the orthodox medicalised process in carrying out the act on their daughters, sisters or any other female for that matter. They should expose in a professional manner the health complications of the practice without condemning the custom of the practicing communities. This should be done by, joining forces with other organizations- human rights groups, law enforcement agents or women groups interested in the abrogation of the practice to expose intransigent perpetrators of the practice within their ranks.

(e) Parents and Socialization of the Child
The family is the first agent of socialization and this entrust the role of the management of the child first with the parents who are the primary agents of transmitting ideas on the child at very early stages in life. Parents should therefore, ensure that children are socialized to see themselves as equals in their own rights performing distinct roles no matter the sex. The issue of sex preference in socialization process should be discouraged. Parents should teach children particularly, the females about sexuality education, and not mystify the concept of sex. This would help equip the adolescent female to cope extensively with the challenges of reproductive health dangers like protective sex, unwanted pregnancies, abortion and the issue of female circumcision that her body is confronted with when she is ignorant.

12.3. Conclusion
One of the major impediments against controlling the poor reproductive health of young people in general, and adolescent females in particular is the lack of awareness of the risk faced by this vulnerable group of the Nigerian population. Hence, the recognition of the existence of the avoidable factors in the majority of teenage maternal deaths must be the first step in designing and implementing reproductive health care programs adequate for young people. The Nigerian government should confront these avoidable factors of socio-cultural and legal impediments by honouring all international resolutions from various conferences, and organizations pertaining women's welfare that she is signatory. Therefore, there should be a global partnership with international organizations to confront the harmful traditional health practices like female circumcision and the issue of illegal abortion that had rendered a large population of adolescent females dead or physically incapacitated.

This study reaffirms the overwhelming importance of educating women and educations direct and indirect influence not only on illegal abortion, and contraceptive use but also on the dangers of female circumcision and the status of women. This research should signal to the Nigerian government and policy makers the urgency of formulating legislations to outlaw female circumcision and liberalize or legalize abortion in the interest of the adolescent females in particular, and women in general. While in the long term, women's education level must be increased, in the short term, strategies such as engaging religious, community and opinion leaders in the National Health Planning Programs must be encouraged. This may help achieve more immediate improvements in discouraging the practice of female circumcision, illegal and dangerous abortion, as well as the administration of dangerous contraceptives by quacks in local communities where traditional and religious norms are used to resist change and improvement in women's reproductive health.

Finally, though adolescent females were more likely than older women to die of maternal causes, parental records indicate in the Nigerian Population Review (1991) 'that adolescents who died were significantly less likely to have been at high risk.' This suggest that policies pertaining to adolescent females health were either not in place or not sufficiently sensitive. Thus a genuine legislation should take into consideration recommendations above for the reproductive health interest of the adolescent female in particular, as it has to do with legislation on abortion and against female circumcision. Furthermore, this researcher anticipates a follow-up study to this work in order to provide a more comprehensive health policy for adolescent females in particular, and adolescents in general in Nigeria.

Appendix I
Biographical Notes of Respondents

Miss Akpo, I

Born in 1985 into a Christian monogamous family in Benin City. She is third in hierarchy among six children. She is from the Itsekiri ethnic group, one of the existing minority ethnic groups in Nigeria. By virtue of her parental background, she is a practicing Christian by faith. Currently, she is in the senior secondary School level, Class 3. Her ethnic group is one of the very few in Nigeria that do not believe in the tradition of female circumcision. Miss Akpo as a practising Christian detests anything that has to do with abortion. She is not circumcised.

Miss Etin, J

Born in 1984 into a polygamous family set up in Sapele. Her father has two wives and fourteen children. Her mother who is the elder of the wives has twelve children, of eight girls and four boys and the second wife has two children. She is from a Christian background and currently attends Zik Grammar School Sapele, where she is in the senior secondary level class three. She hails from the Urhobo ethnic group in Nigeria-the fourth largest in Nigeria. Her ethnic group are staunch believers in the tradition of female circumcision. She condemns abortion because of her Christian religious belief. However, she is a victim of female circumcision.

Miss Efej, M

Born in 1983 in the city of Warri, Delta state. She is from a monogamous and Christian background. Her parents gave birth to five children in a combination of two girls and three boys. She is the third child and second girl in the hierarchy. Presently, she attends Chude Girls' Grammar School Sapele and in the senior secondary class. She is from the Urhobo ethnic group where female circumcision is a known and widely accepted cultural practice. Although, she has not been circumcised at the time of the group discussion, there is a high possibility that she will not escape the exercise, since her elder sister had gone through the surgical knives of trado- medical midwives. She abhors abortion but advocates a legislation that should grant adolescent females the opportunity to seek safe abortion whenever the need arose.

Miss Ugua, O

Born in Sapele town in 1983 into a polygamous setting. Her father had two wives until 1995 when he divorced the second. Her mother was the elder of the two and the only one left at home at the moment. They are ten children in number, made up of eight girls and two boys. She is currently in her senior secondary class at Zik's Grammar school Sapele. She is a Christian by faith and from the Urhobo ethnic group where the practice of female circumcision is a known cultural phenomenon. She was circumcised very early- when she was about 12 years old.

Miss Arie, O

Born in 1983 into a monogamous and Christian family. They are seven children in number, made up of three girls and four boys. She is currently a student in the senior secondary class in the college. She is from the Urhobo ethnic stock where the practice of female circumcision is revered. Although, she was yet to be circumcised she revealed that two of her elder sisters had underwent the process. Her idea on religion also affects her conception on indiscriminate abortion. But she consents to a proposal or legislation to curb and control the practice.

Miss Esth

Born in 1983 in Sapele. She has a Christian and monogamous family background. Her parent has five children, made up of four girls and one male. She hails from the Itsekiri ethnic stock where female circumcision is culturally prohibited. Because of her Christian and family background she detest abortion and strongly condemns the practice of female circumcision by practicing communities. She had just graduated from the senior secondary school level at the time of this interview.

Miss Goll, S

Born in 1982 in Sapele and hail from the Itsekiri speaking ethnic group in Nigeria. Her father has just her mother as a wife and ten children. They are equitably divided, five males and five females. She is from a Christian background and attended both primary and secondary schools in Sapele. Because of her ethnic background she abhors the practice of female circumcision. On abortion, she was reserved but called for mechanisms to control the spate of resultant death from illegally perpetuated abortion.

Miss Uvob, G

Born in 1982 in Sapele to Urhobo parentage. She attended her elementary and secondary schools in the same town of her birth. Her father was a polygamist and had large retinue of wives before his death. Her mother gave birth to five of them and she is the first daughter. Her parents were both illiterates and petty traders, and because of their cultural beliefs on female circumcision she and her immediate younger sister have been victims of the exercise. She admitted the experience was harrowing, and more so, consented to have engaged in illegal abortion for more than once.

Miss Okih, S

Born in Benin City in 1983 to a monogamous and Christian family. They are a family of ten. Her parents gave birth to eight of them, five are females and the other three are males. She hails from the Itsekiri ethnic tribe where female circumcision is outlawed by culture. She was one of the very few who has been exposed to sex education teaching at this level. This is because she attends a private Secondary School that emphasizes on the 'know your health rights.' On the issue of abortion she saw no reason why the practice should not be legalised.

Miss Adib, E

Born on May 17, 1982 in Sapele. Though, she is from a polygamous and Christian oriented family backgrounds, she attends the Saint John's Anglican Church, Amukpe near Sapele. The father who was married to two wives has five children. Both parents of her are separated. Her mother used to be the first wife. She is the first of the five kids. Her mother had two of the five children while the second woman had the remaining three. Her father is a custom officer while her mother a teacher by profession. At the moment, Adib and her younger sister live with their mother. She is currently in the senior secondary class, at Saint Ita's Grammar school, Sapele. She hails from the Urhobo ethnic group where female circumcision is widely practiced. Although, she was yet to be circumcised she claimed that it was just a matter of time she was sure to be. Her mother kept on reminding her of the operation, which is a process of initiation to womanhood or puberty. On abortion issues she holds the view that it is bad because of her Christian orientation, but would support just any scheme that will help to reduce the rate of adolescent females death that result from illegal and dangerously perpetuated abortions of unwanted pregnancies.

Miss Clar O

Born in Sapele on April 5, 1978 and hails from the Urhobo ethnic group in Nigeria. Her father who is late was married to seven wives and had fifteen children. The divide is made up of eight females and seven males. She is number fourteen in the hierarchy of children. Her mother is a petty trader and traditional midwife. Her late father was also a petty trader. She holds very staunch religious beliefs, with strict adherence to the Jehovah Witness faith. Because of her religious belief she condemns outright every act of abortion- legal or illegal and also detest the practice of female circumcision, which to her has no religious or biblical support.

Miss Regi A

Born in 1982 into a polygamous home and hails from Okpe- Urhobo ethnic group in Nigeria where female circumcision is a well-known cultural practice. Her father had two wives and seven children. While the seven children belong to her mother who also is the first of the two wives, the second wife was yet to have children. Her father is a Carpenter by profession and her mother a petty trader. She is also from a Christian family background and attends the Christ Gospel Church. Regi attended Egbo Commercial Grammar School in Kokori where she sat for her school certificate examination and awaiting result at the time of this group discussion.

Miss Imus, B

Born on June 4, 1982 in Sapele and from monogamous background. She hails from Ika-North, where female circumcision is a partial cultural practice. She is the last of six children of her parents and attended Uvwievwe Grammar School at Abraka. Her parents were not well educated. The father works as a Laboratory attendant officer with Eku Baptist hospital and the mother a petty trader. She is a

Christian by faith and worships with the First Baptist Church in Sapele. She was convinced that since all her elder sisters were not circumcised she too would not be circumcised. Her parents are not practitioners of the act in spite of the partial form of its existence in her culture area. She is against illegal abortion and support legislation to control the practice.

Miss Edju, E

Born on August 29, 1978 in Sapele, and from a monogamous background and Christian by faith. Her parent has six children- two of them males, and four females. She could not complete her secondary education because she got pregnant along the line. She had contention with her parents over the issue of her getting circumcised before giving birth, since they hail from the Urhobo ethnic group where female circumcision is held sacred. Though not married, she has a nursing baby boy for the man and claimed to get married to him in the future. Presently, she is engaged in petty provision sales for the upkeep of herself and the baby.

Miss Abdu, R

Born on October 7, 1975 in Kano to Fulani parentage. Her parents were migrants to the southern part of Nigeria in the early 1950s. Though she had all her educational training from primary to the Polytechnic level in the North. She had a terrible experience with the issue of female circumcision and abortion when she was very young and all of these affected her life till date. Though, practicing Moslem by faith, she was of the opinion that the practice of female circumcision in the North was the same with what obtained in the South. Even religion in her words is use to sustain the practice in the north. She holds, that there should be legislation to outlaw the practice of female circumcision, alternatively girls should be given the opportunity to decide whether they wanted it done on them or not. She also believed she would not have had the only child if abortion was legalized.

Miss Okpo, B. G

Born on May 28, 1975 to Dr. and Mrs. Okpo in Sapele. Both parents are orthodox health providers. The father a medical doctor and mother a nursing midwife. She is from the Itsekiri ethnic group in Nigeria, who culturally are not practitioners of female circumcision. She attended the Ambrose Alli University, Ekpoma, where she obtained a degree in Economics. A Christian by faith and worships with the 'Redeem Christian Church of God.' She is the third of eight children, where seven of them are females and one male. She condemns female circumcision but hold that, if the act would threaten the stability of her home in future, she would do it to protect her marriage. On abortion, she supports totally legislation to legalize or liberalize it.

Miss Tolu E

Born in 1973 in Sapele into a monogamous family. They are ten children in number, made up of six females and four males. The father is a trader while the mother a teacher by occupation. Tolu graduated from the University of Benin, where she obtained a degree in Geography and Regional Planning. Tolu's father is from the Urhobo ethnic group, an area where female circumcision is the practice, and while her mother hails from the Itsekiri ethnic group where the practice is culturally prohibited. Interestingly, she is neither circumcised nor any of her sisters. The choice of circumcising or not, is left to them by the parents who understand, that it could be compromised. In her case, the mother influence decided on the circumcision aspect. She swore not to circumcise her female children except when resistance comes from her future husband. On abortion, she supports legislation to legalise it.

Mrs. Imen, R

Born in 1967 at Amukpe near Sapele and hails from the Okpe speaking area of the Urhobo culture. She is married but yet to have children. On passing out from college she went straight for training in health technology. Presently, she works as a local government staff attached to the Ministry of Health, in Sapele. She hails from the female circumcision practicing community and herself passed through the operation from the hands of traditional midwife.

She supports the continuation of the practice but recommends a medicalization of the process of operation. She condemns abortion whether legal or illegal, but recommend that adolescents and women should be educated on their sexuality and encouraged to engage in family planning. Interestingly, Imen is a Christian by faith.

Mrs. Egbo, M

Born in 1956 to illiterate parents and from a polygamous background. She hails from Agbor in Ika- North Local Government Area of Delta State and a Christian by religion. The ethnic group from which she hails are partial practitioners of female circumcision. After her secondary education she enrolled in a commercial institute where she studied secretariat studies. Presently, she is a senior typist with the civil service. Though circumcised, she antagonises the continuous perpetuation of female circumcision, as it has no convincing benefits. On abortion she condemns it outright but call for education of the youths and adolescents to understand reproductive health issues. She is married with three children. She vows not to circumcise the females among them.

Mrs Akep, R

Born in 1954 in the former Okpe division. With a background that is polygamous, and highly traditional, her father was against the concept of women been trained. It took the effort of the mother who was a petty trader to maintain her educational demands. Today, Mrs. Akep who is married into a polygamous setting with eight children is a qualified Professional teacher. She is a Christian practitioner and condemns any form of abortion but discourages the act of female circumcision. She was herself a victim of female circumcision because she hails from a culture area where the practice is held very high. She is a strong advocate for sexual education of adolescents and youths on the issues of reproductive health.

Madam Onem, R

Born in 1936 to Urhobo parents. Her father was an accomplished polygamist with so many wives, and many children. She grew up in a typical traditional setting where the father advocates against the training of women. This is the reason Madam Onem is illiterate today. However, she took to trading like her mother and became successful. Because she was not given the opportunity to be educated, she vowed to educate all of her female children like males. Though she is currently a widow, she has seven children made up of four girls and three males, and all of them educated to certain levels without any preference. With her polygamous experience at both family and marital levels she advices her children to be wary of such practices except when the situation was difficult to control.

She strongly supports the practice of female circumcision and believes in what she called numerous benefits especially 'the curbing of promiscuity' and she condemns the practice of abortion whether legal or illegal and termed it 'murder.' She is however, an active Christian practitioner unlike her parents, and admonished parents to be up to their responsibility of taking adequate care and control of their children.

Mrs Ahia, B

Born about 47 years ago (2000) at Ijenesa village, in Ethiope-East local government area. Although, she is from a polygamous background, but was fortunate to be trained by her father to the level she currently attained for which she was ever grateful. She is married with four children, made up of two males and two females. She trained as an orthodox health provider from the Institute of Health, Benin City in 1982. Though an employee and a senior health officer (i.e. senior nursing sister) at the General Hospital Sapele, she is also a proprietor of a private Maternity and Clinic at Jesse town. She claimed that being an unfortunate victim of female circumcision she would not allow such on her female children. On abortion she advocate the law to legalize it so as to be able to control the spate of illegal abortions perpetuated both by orthodox and unorthodox health providers. Above all, she supports the concept of enlightenment as the major mechanism to awaken the populace awareness to the dangers of female reproductive health. She is a devoted Christian by faith.

Mrs Okpa, R

Born on May 26, 1958 at Okwabude village in Okpe local government area of Delta state to illiterate parents, she strived to acquire western education with the cooperation of her mother who was the second wife in a polygamous marriage. She was the last of four children of her mother. After her primary and secondary education she yearned for more qualifications, which took her to the Petroleum Training Institute, Warri, where she did a family planning course on general health in 1997. Before this time she was already working as an orthodox health provider at the ante- natal department of the Central Hospital Sapele. After her course at the PTI she returned as a senior staff in the unit she was. She is married also into a polygamous system, but unlike her mother she is the eldest of the wives, and she has seven children- two of them are females and five are males. Though, she was circumcised by her parents she regrets the exercise and pledged not to do it to her children no matter the pressure from her husband. On abortion she regrets the trend of unwarranted deaths resulting from adolescent females and call for enlightenment and awareness campaign on reproductive health. She is a renowned orthodox health provider in Sapele Central hospital and a very devoted Christian.

Madam Mak, M

Born in 1934 at Ijenesa, Jesse in Ethiope- East local government area of Delta state and into a typical polygamous set up that was very traditional, she was given surprisingly the opportunity of acquiring western education by her parents but dropped out, because of what she described as "… not clever enough…the inability to cope with the strains of western education." This situation prompted her to take to the trade in trado- medicine since the age of 22, and since then she has put in about 42 years in trado- medical practice. She is a widow with only a surviving son. Despite, the fact that she was circumcised, in the course, of her practice she was at most times a traditional midwife engaged in the circumcision of women because of her belief in 'its benefits.' Today, she is no more engaged in that aspect of the practice because of what she describes as the strains of the practice and her debilitating age which makes it difficult for her to carry out the operation that she describes as 'severe and needs a high level of concentration and attention with good sight.' She however, supports the practice and advocates its continuity, but recommends the medicalization of the process because of the pains that is associated with the traditional methods of circumcision.

She condemns outright the advocate for the liberalization of abortion and call for government to rather promulgate harsh laws to arrest perpetrators and practitioners.

Mrs Adi, V

She is a renowned female trado- medical expert and was born in an Okpe village near Sapele about 42 (2000) years ago. She had the opportunity of attaining some level of education to standard six and later, trained as an auxiliary nurse before retiring to trado-medical practice specializing in the treatment of all forms of women reproductive health illnesses. She combines both orthodox and unorthodox health approaches in her treatment of ailments. She is married with children. She admitted to performing abortions for adolescents and adults alike as well as engage in the practice of female circumcision. Although, she acknowledged the numerous health dangers associated with the practice, she claims that she does it to earn income rather than being convinced on the traditional reasons for the practice. She has no plans of quitting the practice of female circumcision, and perpetuating abortion soon, in spite of her awareness of the health dangers, except when she finds other lucrative means of earning income. Her trado-medical home doubles her residence. Surprisingly, she combines both traditional and Christian faith.

Mrs Muo, S

Born in the late 1940s in the Isoko division of the old Mid-western state. After her secondary education she proceeded to the University to earn a degree in the Social sciences and worked with the public service for over twenty-five years before retiring into active Politics. She is currently one of the three female senators of the 109 members parliament in the fourth republic- the highest law making body in Nigeria. She is married with children and a Christian by faith.

Mrs. Ayat, F

About 44years old and was born in the northern part of Nigeria. She acquired all her education in the North, and worked in the public service before engaging in the politics of the fourth republic. In 1999 she won the election into the lower house of the National Assembly. She is a member of the women committee in the house of representative and a strong advocate for women's rights especially their reproductive health rights. She is married with children and an Islamic adherent by religion and faith.

Master Enak, O

Born in 1985 in Sapele town and from a polygamous background. His father who is an engineer by profession and works with the Shell Petroleum development Company (SPDC) has two wives and six children. Four of them are males and two are females. He hails from the Urhobo speaking area of Delta state and a practicing Christian by faith. Presently, he attends Ufuoma Mixed secondary school Sapele. Though two of his elder sisters were circumcised, he personally does not like the practice. He is in support of legislation against the practice and advocates the same in support of legalization of abortion.

Master Esum, D

Born in Sapele on December 1982, and attended his secondary education in Warri, Delta state. He hails from the Agbor speaking ethnic group of Ika-North local government area of the state. His father is a renowned polygamist with four wives and eleven children. Six of them are males and five are females. The father is the district manager of Uni-Petrol, western division in Nigeria. He is a Christian and does not believe in female circumcision and encourages laws against the practice and laws to legalize abortion. All his sisters were not circumcised and there was no intention on the part of his parents to do that in the nearest future since they hail from an area where the practice is partially practiced.

Master Ibeg, M

Born in 1981 at Sapele, and attended primary and secondary schools in the same town. His father an employee of BIDWELL oil drilling company in Port Harcourt had two wives and ten children. They are six males and four females. He hails from the Ika speaking ethnic stock in Delta state where the practice of female circumcision is optional and family determined. None of his sisters were circumcised and there is no future intention in that direction. Even his father's wives (his mother inclusive) were not circumcised. He is against the culture in practicing communities. Similarly, he advocates legislation to control the practice and to liberalize abortion. He is a practicing Christian.

Master Okev

Born on February 10, 1981 in Sapele. He attended primary and secondary schools in his place of birth. An Urhobo by ethnic and Christian by religion. His father had one wife and nine children. Six of them are females and three are males. Currently his father is a pensioner. Before his retirement he was an employee with the community development office in the local government unit in Sapele. Though he hails from the female circumcision practicing area he condemns the practice as barbaric. Unfortunately, all his sisters had gone through this operation. On abortion he supports the law to liberalize it in order to restore sanity to the tremendous number of deaths that result from illegally perpetuated abortions by quacks and the greatest victims being the adolescent females.

Master Udud, R

Born on February 1, 1981 in Sapele. He attended his primary and secondary schools in the same town. His father had seven wives and eighty-six children. He claims not to even know the number of males or females, but accepted that 'they recognise themselves.' His father was a prominent business man who was engaged in the import and export business. They hail from Jesse town in the Ethiope-East local government area of Delta state, where the practice of female circumcision is also a predominant practice. According to him, a good number of his sisters were already circumcised because it is a matter of culture. Despite all that, he is not in support of the practice. He claimed to have a number of girl friends whom had underwent dangerous illegal abortion and for that purpose he is in support of any law to legalize the practice to prevent the dangers inherent in the practice by quacks. He is a Christian by faith.

Mister Orig, A

Born in 1980 at Oghara in Ethiope-West local government area of Delta state. He dropped out of college because of financial handicap. He decided to learn a trade in Video recording and was employed as an apprentice under 'Prince Ventures and Communication' in Sapele. His father, a security man in BALLO Shell Company has two wives and nine children. Four of them are females and five males. He is very good Christian and advocates strongly against illegal or legal abortion. He claimed, 'that was the reason he decided to allow his girl friend to give birth to an emergent pregnancy which they both were not prepared for.' For him, abortion in any form is murder and against the will of God. On female circumcision, he does not think it is necessary for women to go through it because it is un-biblical, but that if it must be done, then they should medicalize the process in the hospitals rather than do it with traditionalist.

Mister Onjo, K

Born in 1980 in Sapele and had his primary and secondary education in the same town. Though, he hails from Oghara town near Sapele, his parents were migrant to Sapele in the early 1960s. His father, a known polygamist had eight wives and twenty-three children. Nineteen of them are females and four are males. His parents who are both successful traders are both illiterate. The ethnic group of Onjo are staunch practitioners of female circumcision and the parents being traditionalist are very strong faithful of the practice. All of Onjo sisters' are circumcised. He too, believes in the practice and vowed to continue it on his female children. On abortion, he agreed to have perpetuated it more than three times on his chain of girl friends. He is currently a graduate from the college and awaiting result to get into higher institution of learning.

Mr. Farn, O

Born in Sapele town and in his early 30s. He had his primary and secondary education in the same town. His parents who migrated, to Sapele town due to the demands of public service, where his father served, hails from Ethiope-East local government area of Delta state. His father was a retired high ranked customs officer and a polygamist before his death some two years ago (2000). He had three wives and eighteen children. About three of them are females and the rest males. Farn is currently studying for his postgraduate degree at the University of Benin at the time of this interview. He believes in the preservation of the culture of the people but advocate a more civil way of the carrying out female circumcision. He believes that the idea to legalize abortion was good but recommended that an effective mechanism must be put in place to monitor the exercise, so that the process was not abused by adolescents, and the good intention of advocates frustrated. He is a Christian by religion.

Mr. Egbo, J

Born in one of the Okpe villages in 1956 to very poor and illiterate parents. His family background affected his inability to acquire western education. His parents were peasant farmers, and in order to prepare for the survival of the future he learned various forms of trade like the making of craft for survival. Today, he is married with children and doubles by working as a night watchman attached to the school of midwifery in Sapele. He is a staunch believer on female circumcision and admonished any form of abortion whether legal or illegal. He claimed neither to be a strong Christian nor a strong traditionalist. For him he is twisted between the two.

Mr. Fofe, A

Born in 1945. His father hails from Itsekiri ethnic group and the mother Urhobo. Mr Fofe had some basic education to the secondary school level. He is married with a surviving daughter. He is a public servant and salary earner. For him, the issue of female circumcision is unnecessary and should be banned. On abortion, he holds that under whatever guise, it should be frowned at by society. He called for stiff laws to deal with perpetrators, and not to encourage the practice by legalizing it. He called on parents to educate their children properly on issues of sex and reproductive health. Mr. Fofe is a practicing Christian.

Mr. Wede, W

Born in 1930, and an Urhobo by ethnic. Papa Wede as he is popularly called was a renowned Jehovah Witness adherent before he was expelled from the congregation because of what he called his radical ideas of having more than one wife. He has so many children from more than one wife. He is highly educated and retired as an educationist. On retirement, he is a freelance journalist and practitioner. It is his convinced belief that female circumcision has immense benefits and must be continued. He antagonises any idea of legislating against the practice and on the liberalization of abortion. All his female children were circumcised.

Chief Egbe, J

Born in 1923 at Okha village in the present Edo state. Though, his parents descended from the Urhobo ethnic stock. He attempted to acquire western education but opted out after his standard two class for a practice in trado-medicine. He specializes in a wide range of curative- from women reproductive health to traditional acupuncture and mental illness. He has so many wives and many children that he has even lost counts of number. He is a strong advocate of female circumcision, and against any form of abortion. However, he accepted that he has traditional contraceptives to check unwanted pregnancy but can only administer it with the consent of the husband or parents of the young adolescent female. He is a traditional religious worshipper. His private residential home doubles as his trado-medical home. He is assisted, effectively by, both male and female apprentices. Some of his wives and children are also involved in the trade.

Chief Oko

Born in a village called Ovadje in Jesse in 1938 to a polygamist father. His father was married to four wives, and his mother was the third. His father gave birth to fifteen children. Nine of who were males and six others were females. He was the fourth in number of hierarchy of children. Like his parents, he attempted to acquire western education, but failed in his first try and dropped out of school: He then decided to take to the profession of his father who was a successful trado- medical practitioner in his village. He learned as an apprentice under his father before he left to establish his own private practice. In order not to be seen as competing with his father line of trade in the same village, he decided to leave the village to a nearby one to establish. Since then, he has been successful. The death of his father made him to relocate to his place of birth to continue his father heritage.

Chief Oko is married to seven wives and has thirty-two children. Ten of whom are males and the other twenty-two are females. He is an ardent believer of tradition and does not believe in any idea of change. He believes in the continuation of female circumcision and does not encourage any law that would ban the practice and frowns at advocates calling for the legalization of abortion. He rather called on parents to be up to their biddings in taking perfect control of their family and their ward.

Dr. Okun, J

He is in his mid 40s, and the proprietor of Ebony Clinic, a private health concern in Warri. He hails from the Yoruba speaking ethnic group. He had his elementary, and secondary education in the Western part of the country. He attended the University of Ife, Nigeria from where he acquired his degrees in Biochemistry and Medicines. He is married with four children. His wife is a trained orthodox midwife working with the Shell Development Company clinic in Warri. He admonished the continuous practice of female circumcision because of the numerous health dangers and also, advocates for a law to legalize abortion to avoid the patronage of quacks and to reduce the number of adolescent female victims and casualties from such services. He is a practicing Christian by faith.

Barrister Peter, E

Born in 1965 at Ughelli, in Delta state Nigeria and hails from the Urhobo ethnic group. He did his elementary school in Ughelli before proceeding to Saint Peter Clavers College, Aghalokpe and Government College Ughelli to earn his School certificate and A/L certificate respectively. Thereafter, he attended the Universities of Benin, and Ibadan, where he obtained degrees in Sociology and Anthropology, and Law respectively. Later, he went to the University of Lagos where he bagged a Master of Law degree. He is a private legal practitioner and a renowned human right advocate. He is married and a staunch advocate against the tradition of female circumcision calling it a 'cultural violence.' On abortion he calls for effective law to be put in place to check the practice of quacks. He is a Christian by religion.

Hon. Bar. Bala, J

He is in his mid 30s. Born in London and hails from the Okpe speaking ethnic group- one of the dialectic component of the Urhobo tribe. His parents are well educated and he is a beneficiary of this veritable educational legacy. He studied Law at the University of Ekpoma, Nigeria before proceeding to engage in private legal practice. He went into Politics thereafter. Today, he is a honourable member, of the House of Assembly in Delta State. Because of his principled stance he had to resign his position as the Chief Whip of the house of assembly, and opted to be at the background. In spite of that, he is a force of recognition and voice not to undermine in the present house of assembly. He is a member of numerous committees of the house. He is married with children, and of the view that the health implication of female circumcision was enough grounds for the house to legislate against the practice. On abortion, he contends that effective law should be promulgated to save adolescent females from the abuse of quacks. He is a Christian by faith.

Dr. Beid, G

He is in his early 50's. Born in Edo state and had a very strong educational foundation by his parent. After his elementary education he went straight to the university to study medicine. Before entering into politics of the fourth republic he ran his private clinic in Benin-city, he is presently a member of the House of Representative, and the chairman of the house committee on health.

He is married and has children. His wife hails from the Itsekiri ethnic speaking group where female circumcision is culturally disallowed. She is a trained midwife and works with the University of Benin Teaching Hospital (UBTH), Nigeria. Dr. Bied is a Christian by faith.

Appendix II
Focus Group Discussion, Case Study and Personal Interview Guide on Adolescent Females Reproductive Health in Nigeria: A study on the legislation and socio-cultural impediments to Abortion and against Female Circumcision in Nigeria.

A. Introduction
- **Welcome to this interview / discussion.**

The purpose of this research is to highlight the problems associated with the increase in the spate of unwanted pregnancies, abortions contraception, and poor accessibility to contraceptives in our society; as well as, government poor attitude of non-compromise, by making it illegal for women to embark on abortion / contraception. This is further enhanced, by our own effective socio-cultural systems.

Also, the tacit support of government and by extension socio-cultural processes towards the perpetuation of Female Genital Mutilation (FGM), and their poor attendance to the AIDS/HIV crises in Nigeria forms a fundamental basis for the importance of this research and interview.

Thus, the findings from this study would be purposefully, directed at addressing most of the shortcomings at both the individual, organizational and governmental levels concerning the advocacy, and formulation of uniform and positive policies towards these vital reproductive health issues, especially as it affects the women

- **Open expressions of opinions welcome.**
- Tape recorder will be used to allow retrieval of information. For anonymous purpose and confidentiality, do not mention your name before responding to the issues raised.

B. Bio-Data Issues (Biography of respondents)
- When and where were you born?
- Tell me about your family background?
  - -How many are you in number?
  - -What is your / their educational background?
  - -Your / their religious beliefs?
  - -Your / their occupational backgrounds?
  - -What is the form of marriage contracted by your parents?
  - -What about you?
- How would you describe your relationship with your family?
- Do you have friends?
  - -What is your relationship with your friends?
  - -Do you have boy / girl friend?
  - -How did you meet him or her?
  - -Tell me briefly about him or her?

C.   Premarital sex
-    Perception\ Conceptualization of sex.
-    Terms used for sex.
-    Who should have sex\ complete run\ a bang?
-    Differentiate between girl friends and babies or 'wife'.
-    How do you view sex before marriage?
-    What is the right age to start sex?
-    What are your reservations?
-    What do you say about the sexual behaviour of adolescents \ youths,

     your age group ?

D.   Pregnancy and its outcomes
-    Is pregnancy common among your group?
-    What often happens to such pregnancy?
-    Have you ever had one?
-    Who did you tell first about it?
-    What happened to it / what did you do to get rid it of it?
-    What method did you use to get rid of it?
-    Do you know about girls not seeing their monthly periods?
-    What do they do to induce \ get it?
-    Who advises them on what and where to go?
-    Who would they tell first when it happens?
-    What are the methods you know that are used to induce periods?
-    What about the complications that may arise?
-    How are they handled?
-    Do you know of deaths resulting from such acts?
-    What is \ are responsible?
-    What can be done to reduce the number of abortions / deaths resulting from abortions?
-    What do you think the government should do about the problem?

E. Contraception
-   Level of knowledge: Do you know of the need to prevent pregnancy and infections?
-   What methods \ techniques are known?
-   Are they in use among your age group?
-   Where are they obtained?
-   Who advises you on prevention of pregnancy and infections from sex?
-   What are the obstacles to obtaining contraceptives?
-   What can be done?
-   Is it necessary or not?
-   Present samples of contraceptive here (by the researcher)
-   Reasons for use \ advising the use of contraceptives.

- Reasons for not using or advising the use of Contraceptive
- Would you talk about sex with your parents?
- Reasons why you will?
- Reasons why you will not?
- Who would you discuss sex with?
- Who would you discuss any infection or illness with?
- What about illness arising from sex, e.g. gonorrhoea?

F.   Legislation (Policy) and Contraception \ Abortion
- Are you aware of obstacles preventing youths \ adolescents from obtaining contraceptives in public hospitals or any where ?
- What are your reactions?
- What do you know about abortion in Nigeria? legal or illegal?
- Who told you about what you know?
- What do you think about the laws on abortion? (State them here)
- Are they necessary? What are your reasons?
- What are your views on liberalizing these laws? And, how?
- How do we change attitude to liberalizing these laws?

G. Health Behaviour
i) Female Genital Mutilation (FGM).
- Are you circumcised? / What were your experiences during FGM?
- At what age were you circumcised?
- Who carried out the circumcision?
- How many of you in your family are circumcised?
- About how many of your friends do you know are circumcised?
- What are the reasons for circumcising females / males?
- What do you think are the dangers associated with FGM?
- Do you think, it is still necessary to carry out FGM?
- If no, why? If yes, why?
- How do you think FGM could be discouraged?
- What other contributions would you like to make towards the current debate on discouraging FGM?

ii) Sexually Transmitted Diseases (STD's).
- Have you ever heard of sexually transmitted disease (STD)?
- If yes, indicate which of the STD's you know or have heard of, or even contracted?
- Do you know of anyone who has or has had a STD?
- If yes, what is the person to you?
- Indicate how you / others have been treated from STD's.
- What do you know about the causes of STD'?
- How are other STD's excluding AIDS transmitted?

iii) AIDS / HIV.
- Have you ever heard about AIDS?
- What do you know are the causes of AIDS?

- Who told you about what you know?
- Do you know anyone who has been treated of AIDS?
- If yes, what is the person to you?
- Have your sexual behaviour been modified since learning of AIDS
- If yes, how? and, to what extent?
- How would you describe the sexual behaviours of youths now?
- What do you think could be done by the individual, organizations (NGO's in particular) and governmental agencies to check the problems of AIDS / HIV amongst youths and adults in our society?

H) Other Cultural Issues
- What are some of the cultural taboos relating to sex that you know?
- Can you outline some of the traditional methods for the protection of the individual against AIDS/HIV, STD's etc.
- What is the impact of your religion on the issues of abortion, the use of contraceptives, as well as on the issue of sex generally? What does it also, speaks about the AIDS/HIV diseases? How are infected persons that you know treated in your congregation?
- What are some of the enlightenment channels to sensitise people on the problems of these crucial reproductive health issues that you know? Can you also, identify some of the traditional enlightenment methods as well? Which of these channels do you think are more effective?
- Is there anything, we have not discussed / asked that you would like to say?
- Is there anything you would like to ask or get more information on? Please feel free to do so.
  Thank You So Much For This Discussion / Interview.

Appendix III
Transcription Notations.
1. Participants / Respondents
I   = Interviewer
A-Z= Alphabets representing the first names of respondents / participants.
2. Pause
(…): Short pause or talking pause- took about two to three seconds.
(……): Long pause- for trying to recall memory, or thinking of what to say. This normally was more than five seconds.
3. Exclamations
 For example, Oh! eh !: exclamation for the affirmation of an idea or to show surprise
4. Double use of words
For example, no! no! or yes! Yes!: indicates emphasis on the subject or issue of discussion
5. **Words in Italics**: Indicate emphasis
6. /: Change of the topic or an introduction of a new idea, point or issue
7. --: Indicate incomplete statements
8. **(cut in):** Interruption as a result of anger or being impatient with the point raised by other participants or the interviewer's question
9. **Parenthesis**: Sudden outburst like (laughing aloud), (shouting), (anger), (unclear issues) etc. are shown in parenthesis or brackets
10. A new line starts with a change of the speaker

Appendix IV
Abbreviations
AHI   Action Health Initiative
AIDS   Acquired Immune Deficiency Syndrome
ANC   African National Congress
ATP   African Timber and Plywood
BBC   British Broadcasting Corporation
CARAL   California Abortion Rights Action League
CIA   Criminal Investigation Agency
CPS   Contraceptive Prevalence Study
CRLP   Centre for Reproductive Law and Policy
DAAD   Deutscher Akademischer Austauschdienst
D & C   Dilation and Curettage
DHS   Demographic Health Survey
FC   Female Circumcision
FCI   Family Care International
FGE   Female Genital Elongation
FGM   Female Genital Mutilation
FRH   Family Reproductive Health
FU   Freie Universität
FWCW   Fourth World Conference on Women
GADA   Gender and Development Action
GDP   Gross Domestic Product
HB   Health Bill
HIV   Human Immunodeficiency Virus
ICHR   International Conference on Human Rights
ICPD   International Conference on Population and Development
IFPP   International Family Planning Perspectives
IMF   International Monetary Fund
IWHC   International Women's Health Coalition
JHU   John Hopkins University
KAP   Knowledge, Attitude and Practice

KNIECSS Kenya National Information, Education, and Communication

         Situation Survey

MFAD   Ministry of Foreign Affairs- Danida

MYWO   Maendeleo Ya Wanawake Organization

NCPD   National Council for Population and Development

NCWS   National Council for Women Society

NGOs   Non Governmental Organizations

NPR   National Population Review

NSAM	National Survey of Adolescent Males
NSFG	National Survey of Family Growth
OAU	Organization of African Unity
PANA	Pan African News Agency
PATH	Path for Appropriate Technology in Health
PCS	Population Communication Services
PLA	Participatory Learning and Action
PPF	Planned Parenthood federation
PPFA	Planned Parenthood Federation of America
PRB	Population Reference Bureau
PTI	Petroleum Training Institute
SIECUS	Sexuality Information and Education Council of the United States
SOGON	Society of Gynaecology and Obstetrics of Nigeria
STDs	Sexuality Transmitted Diseases
UN	United Nations
UNFPA	United Nations Population Fund
UNGA	United Nations General Assembly
UNICEF	United Nations Children's Fund
USA	United States of America
UTI	Urinary Track Infection
WEL	Women's Electoral Lobby
WHARC	Women's Health and Action Research Centre
WHO	World Health Organization
WHON	Women Health Organization of Nigeria
WIN	Women in Nigeria
WRP	Women's Right Project
YRBS	Youth Risk Behaviour Study

Appendix V
The Map of the Federal Republic of Nigeria showing the 36 states and the
federal capital at the Centre and other Health Information as it affects
adolescents and the girl child.

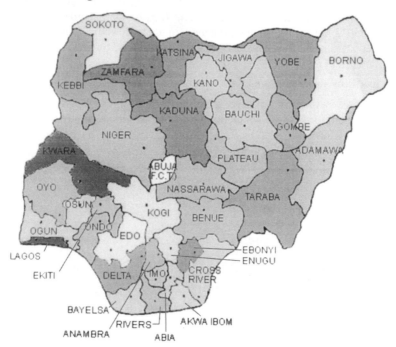

States and their Capital
Abia (Umuahia), Adamawa (Yola), Akwa Ibom (Uyo), Anambra (Awka),
Bauchi (Bauchi), Bayesa (Yenogoa), Benue (Makurdi), Bornu (Maiduguri),
Cross Rivers (Calabar), Delta (Asaba), Ebonyi (Abakaliki), Edo (Benin City),
Ekiti (Ado-Ekiti), Enugu (Enugu), Gombe (Gombe), Imo (Owerri), Jigawa
(Dutse), Kaduna (Kaduna), Kano (Kano), Katsina (Katsina), Kebbi (Birnin
Kebbi), Kogi (Lokoja), Kwara (Ilorin), Lagos (Ikeja), Nassarawa (Lafia), Niger
(Minna), Ogun (Abeokuta), Ondo (Akure), Oshun (Oshogbo), Oyo (Ibadan),
Plateau (Jos), Rivers (Port-Harcourt), Sokoto (Sokoto), Taraba (Jalingo), Yobe
(Adamawa), Zamfara (Gusau)
Area: **923,850 sq km**   Capital: **Abuja.**
Population: **120.8 million, 133 per sq. km, 255% growth**
Life Expectancy: **53** Infant Mortality: **760 per thousands**
Doctors per million: **210.**
Currency: **Naira = 100 kobo (NGN)**

Minors and Adolescents

•Nigeria, children under 15 years of age constitute approximately 43 percent of the population.

Recent estimates indicate that the adolescent fertility rate stands at 115 births per 1,000 women aged 15-19. In 1999, the median age at first birth was estimated at 20 years. Recent reports maintain that at least 50 percent of girls and women have undergone FC/FGM.

Contraception and Abortion

- Currently, an estimated 15 percent of married women report using a family planning method; of these, 9 percent report use of a modern method.

- Studies in 1998 estimated that women in Nigeria obtained abortions at a rate of 25 per 1,000 women aged 15-44; an estimated 60 percent of these, were performed by non-physician providers

Source: The World Bank, World Development Indicators (2000: 39)

Appendix VI

Common Modern Drugs and Local Abortificients mixed and used for Abortion.

1. Codeine or Bee-Codeine Tablets
2. Tetracycline Capsules
3. Andrew Liver Salt Laxative
4. M and B Tablets
5. Guinness Stout Beer
6. Gin: Local or Foreign Brewed
7. Cowries
8. Plantain
9. Native Chalks
10. Ground Pepper
11. Pap
12. Black Native Chalk
13. Potash
14. Lime
15. Tobacco Leaves
16. Ginger Pepper
17. Boundary Tree

Appendix VII

Local and Modern Materials used for Female Circumcision

1. Scissors
2. Razor Blade
3. Sharp stones
4. Small Knives
5. Sharp Broken Bottles

Appendix VIII

Local Substance used for Perpetuating Crude, Dangerous and Illegal Abortions amongst Adolescent Females'. This is normally combined or mixed with modern drugs for medication purpose.

Picture 1: Boundary Tree. The latex is used for abortion.

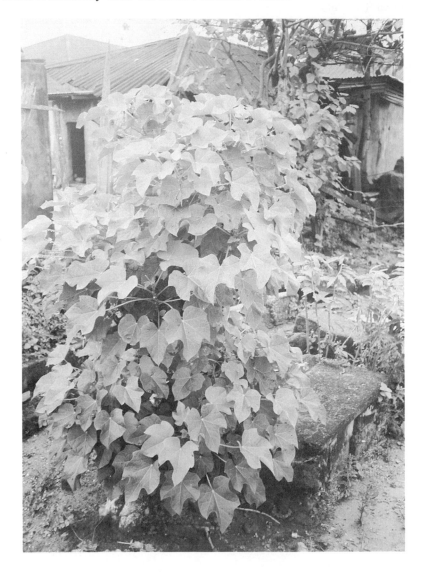

Appendix IX

Some cross sectional photos of participants in focus group, personal interviews and case study sessions.

Pictures 1 and 2: Adolescent males' and females' in focus group discussion.

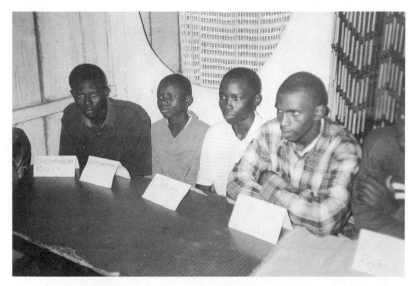

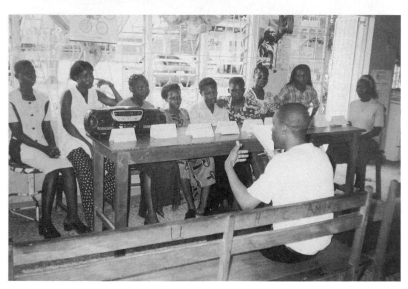

Pictures 3 and 4: Adults and adolescent females' (not in school).

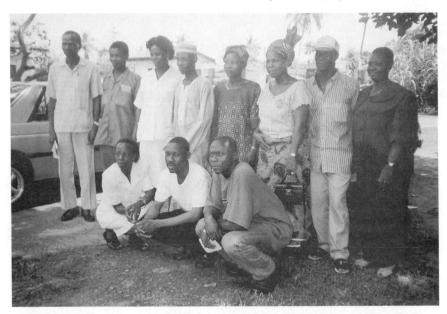

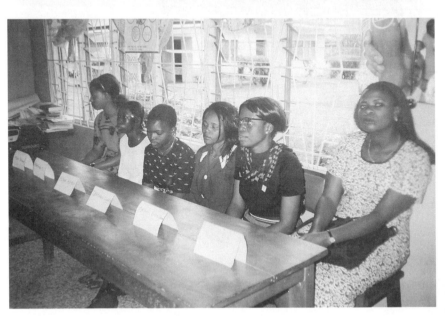

Pictures 5 and 6: Trado- medical health experts (female and male) during personal interview sessions.

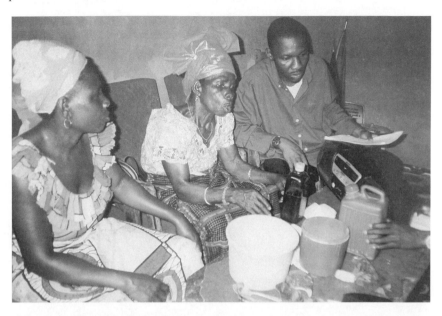

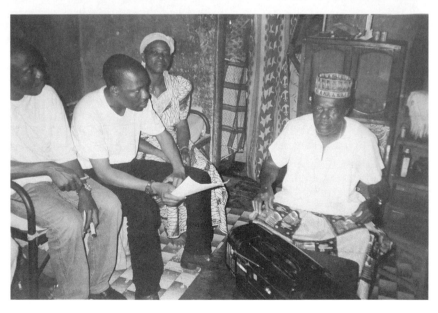

Pictures 7 and 8: Orthodox female health expert and one of my case study interviewee.

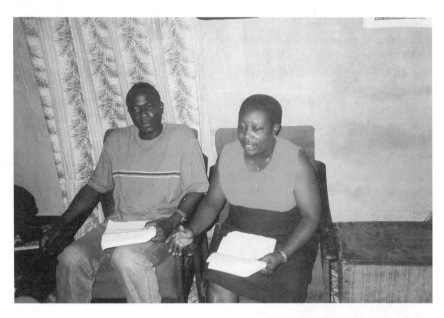

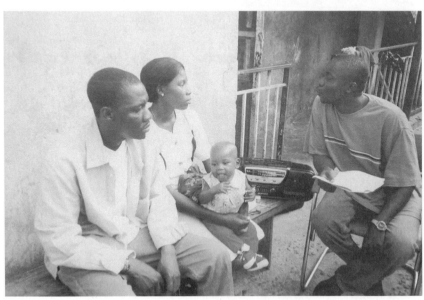

Bibliography /References

Adetoro, O.O. (1986), 'Sceptic induced abortion at Illorin Nigeria: An increasing Gynaecological problem in developing countries' *Asia-Oceania Journal of Obstetrics and Gynaecology,* Vol. 12(2), Pgs. 102-105

----------, (1989), 'A 15-year study of illegally induced abortion mortality at Illorin, Nigeria.' *International Journal of Gynaecology and Obstetrics*, Vol. 29, Pgs. 65-72

Adetoro, O. et al. (1991), 'Socio-Cultural Factors in Adolescent Septic Illicit Abortions at Illorin, Nigeria.' *African Journal of Medicine and Medical Sciences*, Vol. 20(2), Pgs 149 –153

Adetunji, J. (1996), 'Preserving the Pot and the water: A traditional concept of reproductive health in a Yoruba community, Nigeria.' *Social Science and Medicine,* Vol. 43(11), Pgs. 1561-1567

Adewole, I. F. (1992), 'Trends in post-abortal mortality and morbidity in Ibadan, Nigeria', *International Journal of Gynaecology and Obstetrics,* Vol, 38(2), Pgs. 115-118

Adewole, I.F. (1993/1994), 'That our women may live.' *The Nigerian Family Practice*, Vol. 3(2), Pgs. 9-11

African [Banjul] Charter on Human and People's Rights, Organization of African Unity (O.A.U.) Doc. CAB/LEG/67/3/Rev. 5 (1981) (entered into force Oct. 21, 1986)

African Concord. (1991), 'This child must die: Government insists on abortions, and interest groups React' 21 Oct., Pg. 30

AGI Magazine (1998) 'Into A New World: Young Women Sexual and Reproductive Lives.' New York U.S.A

----------, (1999) 'Sharing Responsibility: Women, Society and Abortions Worldwide.' *Daily Champion,* Lagos Pg. 15

Akande, J.O. (1982), "The Constitution of the Federal Republic of Nigeria, with Annotations." London: Sweet and Maxwell.

Akingba, J.B. (1971). "The Problem of Unwanted Pregnancies in Nigeria Today" Akingba Pub. Lagos.

Akumadu, T. (1997), Supra note 15, in the Centre for Reproductive Law and Policy file. March 12, Pages 9-15

Alcorn, R. (1992) "Pro Life Answers to Pro Choice Arguments." Multnomah Books.

Allan G. H. et al, (1998). 'Reproductive mishaps and Western Contraception: An African challenge to fertility theory.' *Population and Development Review,* Vol. 23(3)

Alubo, O. (1999/2000), "The challenges of adolescent sexuality and reproductive health in Nigeria." Research paper no. 166, Takemi Program in International Health, Harvard School of Public Health, Boston U.S.A, Pgs. 1-25

Amin, S. (1972), 'Underdevelopment and Dependency in Black Africa – Origins and Contemporary Forms.' *The Journal of Modern African Studies*, Vol.10 (4), Pgs. 503- 524

Amrita, B. (1995) "The Challenge of Local Feminisms: Women's Movements in Global Perspective" West-view Press, Inc

Arbesman, M. et al. (1993), 'Assessment of the impact of female circumcision on the Gynaecological, genitourinary and obstetrical health problems of women from Somalia: Literature Review and Case Studies.' *Women Health,* Vol. 20, Pgs. 27-42

Armstrong, Sue. (1991) 'Female Circumcision: Fighting a Cruel Tradition.' *New Scientist,* Vol. 2(2), Feb., Pgs. 42-47

Babatunde, E. (1998), "Women's Rites versus Women's Rights: A Study of Circumcision among the Ketu, Yoruba of South Western Nigeria." Africa World Press,

Bailey, P.E. et al. (1988), 'A hospital study of illegal abortion in Bolivia.', *Bulletin of the Pan American Health Organization*, Vol. 22(1), Pgs. 27-41

Barchar, J. (1999), 'Controversy Brew Over Abortion Issues', *Pan African News Agency* (PANA) Feb., Dakar Senegal; Pgs. 1-6

Barker, G. & Fontes, M. (1996), 'Review and Analysis of International Experience with Programmes Targeted on At-Risk Youths.' *Unpublished Report for the Government of Colombia.* World Bank.

Barker, G. & Rich, S. (1992). 'Influences on Adolescent Sexuality in Nigeria and Kenya: Findings from Recent Focus-Group Discussions.' *Studies in Family Planning,* Vol. 23(3)

Beißwenger, K.D., & Höpfner, C. (1993), (eds.) „AIDS FORUM D.A.H. BAND XII: Aspects Of AIDS and AIDS-HILFE", Berlin Pg. 76

Bellew, R.T and King, E. M. (1993), 'Educating Women: Lessons from Experience' in E. M. Kings and M. Hill (Eds.) "Women's Education in Developing Countries, Barriers Benefits and Policies." Baltimore: Published for the World Bank-John Hopkins University Press. Pg. 285

Brabin et al, (1995), 'Reproductive Tract Infections and Abortion among Adolescent Girls in Rural Nigeria.' *The lancet.* Pg. 345

Bradbury R.E. & Lloyd, P. C. (1957), "Ethnographic Survey of Africa" (ed.) By Daryll Forde, 'West Africa Part XIII'. London international African Institute.

Brady, M. (1999), 'Female Genital Mutilation: Complications and Risk of HIV Transmission.' *In AIDS patients care and STDs,* Vol. 13 (12), Pgs. 709-716

Briggs L.A. (1994), 'Post primary school teachers, viewpoint on reproductive health and contraceptive practice among school girls in Port Harcourt, Nigeria.' *Journal of the Royal of the Society of Health,* Vol. 114 (5), Pgs. 235-239

----------, (1998) 'Parents 'viewpoint on Reproductive Health and Contraceptive Practice among Sexually Active Adolescents in the Port Harcourt Local Government Area of Rivers State, Nigeria' *Journal of Advanced Nursing,*

Location: SNDT Church gate. Vol. 27. Pgs. 261-266

Briggs, N.D. (1993), 'Illiteracy and maternal health; educate or die.' *Lancet*, Vol. 341 (8852), Pgs. 1063-1064

Broschüre Zur Ausstellung: Weibliche Genitalverstümmelung, Künstlerinnen und Künstler aus Nigeria Klagen an. Im Stadthaus Mannheim, (2000), Feb. 4, Pgs. 4-36

Burkart, G. (1983), ,Zur Mikroanalyse Universitärer Sozialisation im Medizinstudium: Eine Anwendung der Methode der objektiv-hermeneutischen Textinterpretation' *In: Zeitschrift für Soziologie,* Jg. 12, Heft 1. Pgs. 24-48

Calder, B. et al. (1993), 'Female circumcision / genital mutilation: Culturally sensitive care.' *Health Care Women International,* Vol. 331, Pgs. 712-716

Caldwell, J. C. et al. (1992.), 'Fertility Decline in Africa: A New Type of Transition?' *Population and Development Review*, Vol. 18(2), Pgs. 211 - 242

----------, (1999), 'The Bangladesh fertility decline: an interpretation', *Population And Development Review*, Vol. 25(1): Pgs. 67-68

Caldwell, P. And Caldwell, J. (1987), 'Fertility Control as Innovation: A Report on In-depth Interviews in Ibadan, Nigeria.' *in The Cultural Roots of African Fertility Regimes*. Ed. Van de Walle, E. and Ebigbola, J. Philadelphia: Univ. of Pennsylvania, Pgs. 233 - 251

Calhoun, C. et al, (1994), "Sociology", Sixth Edition, McGraw Hill, Inc

CEDPA/UNFPA (1998), 'From Challenge to Consensus: Adolescents Reproductive Health in Africa.' (CRLP-1995), *'Reproductive Freedom News',* Feb. 10. Vol. IV (3)

Chandrasckhar, S. (1974), "Abortion in a Crowded World: The Problem of Abortion with Special reference to India", London: G. Allen and Unwin

Chapel-Hill, C. (1990), 'Demographic Survey and Nigerian Women', *in Signs* 15(2), Pgs. 259 –284

Chaturachinda, K. et al, (1981), 'Abortion: an epidiomologic study at Ramthibodi Hospital, Bangkok' *Studies in Family Planning,* Vol. 12, Pgs. 257 261

Chege, N.J. et al. (2001), "Assessment of the alternative rights approach for encouraging abandonment of female genital mutilation in Kenya" A report funded and submitted to USAID. Pgs. 1-39

Chen, L.C. et al. (1981), 'Sex bias in the family allocation of food and Health care in rural Bangladesh', *Population and Development Review*, Vol. 7(1), Pgs. 55-70

Chen, P. et al (1982), 'The Dilemma of Parenthood: A study of the value of Children in Singapore.' *The institute of South-East Asian studies*

Children Convention. Article 24 (f), UN-DOC. 1990, A / 44 /49

Cohen, B. and Trussell, J. (1996), eds. 'Preventing and Mitigating AIDS in Sub Saharan Africa: research and Data Priorities for the Social and Behavioural Sciences. Panel on Data and Research Priorities for Arresting AIDS in Sub Saharan Africa.' *National Research Council,* Washington, DC; National

Academy Press

Convention on the Rights of the Child, (1989) General Assembly Resolution 44/25 U.N. GAOR, 44th Sess., Supp. No. 49, at 166, U.N. Doc A/44/49

Cook, R. et al, (1985), "Women: Progress Toward Equality", Wallchart London: International Planned Parenthood Federation

Criminal Code, Laws of the Federation of Nigeria (1958), Volume ii (Cap 42), sections 228-230; 297; and Laws of Northern Nigeria (1963) Penal Code (Cap. 89) sections 232 -234.

David, H.P. (1981) "Abortion Policies in Abortion and Sterilization: Medical and Social Aspects" J.E. Hodgson, ed., Grune and Stratton, New York

Davis, B.O. et al. (1985), "Conceptual Human Physiology", Charles E. Merrill Publishing Company.

Dawit, S. and Mekuria, S. (1993), 'The West Just Doesn't Get It.' *New York Times*, Dec. 7. Pg. 27

Demographic and Health Survey - Sudan. (1989-1990). Calverton, MD: Macro International Inc. Pgs. 115- 118

Demographic and Health Survey - Egypt. (1995). Calverton, MD: Macro International Inc. Pg. 171

Desrosiers, R.C. (1986), 'Origin of the Human AIDS Virus.' *Nature* Vol. 319, Pg. 728

Desilet, A. (1999): 'More Abortions in Canada', *in Awake Magazine*, Feb. 28, Pg. 28

Devereux, George (1954) 'A Typological Study of Abortion in 350 Primitive, Ancient and Pre-industrial Societies', *in Therapeutic Abortion*, ed. Harold Rosen, New York: The Julian Press Inc.

----------, (1955), "A Study of Abortion in Primitive Societies" New York: Julian Press.

Dewane, F. (1999), 'Everyone Right to Life', in Daily Catholic news and views from Catholic Perspective, Catholic World News and Church News at Noticias Eclesiales. Vol. 10(29) Pgs. 8-9

Diggory, P. et al. (1970), "Abortion" London: Cambridge University Press.

Dirie, M.A. & Lindmark, G. (1992), 'The Risk of Medical Complications after Female Circumcision.' *In East African medical journal*, Vol. 69(9), Pgs. 479 482

Djerassi, C. (1979), "The Politics of Contraception: The Present and the Future". New York, G.W. Norton and Company.

Dorkenoo, E. (1995), "Cutting the Rose: female genital mutilation, the practice and its prevention" Minority Rights Group, London.

Douglas, M. (1966), 'Magic and Miracle', *in Purity and Danger: An Analysis of Concepts of Pollutions and Taboo,* London: Routledge & Kegan Paul.

Duffy, J. (1989), 'Clitoridectomy: A nineteenth Century Answer to masturbation.' Presented at The First International Symposium on Circumcision, Anaheim, California, Mar. 1-2, Pgs. 1-4

Egan, T. (1993). 'An Ancient Ritual and a Mother's Asylum Plea.' *New York Times*, Mar. 4, Pg. A25

El Saadawi, Nawal, (1980), "Hidden Face of Eve: Women in the Arab World." Zed Books, London

Ellwood, D.T. (1989), 'The Origin of Dependency, Choices, Confidence or Culture?' *in FOCUS*, Vol. 12, Number 1 Spring and Summer, Pgs. 3-13

Egunjobi G., (1998), 'Catching (and killing) them young' *in THE GUARDIAN*, Sept. 5 (Women And Family Column.) Nigeria. Pg. 30

----------, (1998): 'Death and the Mothers', *in THE GUARDIAN*, Aug. 22, Pg. 10

----------, (1999), 'Cause of a Deadly Scourge', *in THE GUARDIAN*, Dec. 25

Elson, D. (1991), "Male Bias in the Development Process", New York St, Martins Press

Ekwy, P.U. (1997), 'Human Rights and The Women Question', *in THE GUARDIAN*, Mar. 23. Pg. B9

Engle, K. (1992). 'Female Subjects of Public International Law: Human Rights and the Exotic Other Female.' *New England Law Review*, Vol. 26, Pgs. 1509 1526

Enwemnwa, I. (1995), 'Introduction to Social Psychology II', Unpublished Monograph for 200 level Sociology Students, University of Benin, Benin City, Nigeria. Pgs. 1-7

Erikson, E. (1950), 'Childhood and Society.' New York: Norton. In Craig et al, "Sociology", (1994).

Estes, Richard J. (1992), 'Women and Development', an excerpt form Richard J. Estes 1992 "Internationalising Social Work Education: A Guide to Resources for a new Century" Philadelphia: University of Pennsylvania School of Social Work.

Fakayode, E. O. (1977), "The Nigerian Criminal Code Companion." Ethiope Publishing Corporation.

Fariyal, F. et al, (2001), 'what influences Contraceptive use among young women in urban squatter settlements of Karachi, Pakistan?' *In International Family Planning Perspectives*, Sept. edition, Vol. 27(3) Pgs. 130-135

Federal Office of Statistics (Nigeria) and IRD/Macro International Nigeria, Demographic & Health Survey 1990, Columbia, Maryland: IRD/Macro International, 1992

Ferguson, A. (1988), 'School girl pregnancy in Kenya: report of a study of discontinuation rates and associated factors.' 2nd Edition, Nairobi, Kenya, Ministry of Health, Division of Family Health, GTZ Support Unit, Pg. 74

Fitzsimmons, E. (1998), 'Infant Head Moulding: A Cultural Practice.' *Archives Family Medicine*, Vol. 7 (1), Pgs. 88-90

Fletcher, L. et al. (1994), 'Human Rights Violations Against Women.' *Whittier L. Review* Pgs. 336-417

Forde, D. (1951), 'The Yoruba Speaking Peoples of South-Western Nigeria.'

Ethnographic Survey of Africa, London: International African Institute.

FORUM (2000), 'Promoting Post-Abortion Care in Nigeria.' *In A Publication of the Women's Health and Action Research Centre,* Benin City, Nigeria, Vol. 5, no. 1, ISSN: 11118-485X1

FORWARD. (1993), 'Report of the First Study Conference of Genital Mutilation of Girls, in Europe /Western World.' London,

Francone, C. (1984), "Abortion Freedom: A Worldwide Movement". London: George Allen And Unwin.

Free, M.J. (1985), "Condoms: the rubber remedy In Fertility Control", Corson, S.C., Derman, R.J., Tyrer, L.B. (eds.), Boston: Little Brown and Co.

Freud, S. (1947), 'The Ego and the Id" London: Hogarth Press. In Craig et al, "Sociology" (1994).

Gaelesiwe, L. (1999), 'Let's Talk About Sex', *The International Development Magazine,* Issue 6, Second Quarter Pgs. 26-27

Gatara, H.T. and Muriuki, P.W. (1985), 'Project report on Youth Education and Services for Health and Family Life: Summary of situation analyses and Consultation (Nairobi) and Geneva, International Planned Parenthood Federation. African Region, and World Health Organization, Sept. Mimeo Pg. 41

Gather, C. (1996), "Konstruktionen von Geschlechterverhältnissen: Machtstrukturen und Arbeitsteilung bei Paaren im Übergang in den Ruhestand." Berlin: Ed. Sigma. ISBN 389404-416-0.

Giwa-Osagie, O. (2000), ' Women More At Risk', *in The Vanguard*, Jan. 27

Golara, M., Morris, N., & Gordon, H. (1998), 'Prevention of genital tract trauma during labour and delivery in an African population following female genital mutilation.' *Journal of Obstetrics & Gynaecology,* Vol. 18, Pgs. 49-51

Gormick, V. & Barbara, K. (1972), (eds.) "Women In Sexist Society: Studies in power and Powerless", Basic Books Inc.

Granja, A.C. et al. (2001), 'Adolescent maternal mortality in Mozambique', *Journal of Adolescent Health*, 28(4), Pgs. 303-306

Greer, G. (1999). "The Whole Woman", Doubleday, ISBN: 0385 60016X.

Gyepi-Garbrah, B. (1985), "Adolescent Fertility in Nigeria", Boston, MA: Pathfinder Fund.

Hall, G. Stanley, (1981), 'Adolescence: Its Psychology and Its Relations to Physiology, Anthropology, Sociology, Sex, Crime, Religion and Education' (2 vols.) Norwood,

P.A: Telegraph Books, In Craig et al, "Sociology", (1994).

Heath, S. (1982), "The Sexual Fix" New York: Schocken.

Henry, P.D. (1978), "Abortion in Psychological Perspective: Trends in trans national research." New York: Springer Pub.

Henshaw S.K. et al. (1998) 'The incidence of induced abortion in Nigeria' *International Family Planning Perspective,* Vol. 24, Pgs. 156-164

----------. (1999), 'The incidence of abortion worldwide', *International Family*

Planning Perspectives, Vol. 25 (supplement), Pgs. 30-38

Hilgers, et al. (1981), 'Fertility Problems following an Aborted First Pregnancy.' *In new Perspectives on Human Abortion* edited by S. Lembrych, University Publication of America, Pgs. 128-134

Hill and Wang, (1970), "American Friends Service Committee: Who shall live? Mans Control over birth and death; A report Prepared For American Friends Committee Services." New York.

Hosken, F.P. (1989), 'Female Genital Mutilation: Strategies for Eradication'. Paper presented at the first international symposium on circumcision, Anaheim, California, Mar. 1-2, Pgs.3-8

----------, (1993), "The Hoskins Report: Genital and sexual mutilation of Females.' 4th Reviewed Edition. Lexington, Massachusetts, Women's International Network News (WIN)

Hrdy, D. B. (1987), 'Cultural Practices Contributing to the Transmission of Human Immunodeficiency Virus in Africa.' *In review of infectious diseases,* Vol. 9(6), Pgs. 1109-1119

Hrdy, S. B. (1981), "The Woman that Never Evolved", Cambridge, Mass: Harvard University Press

Huntemann, N. B. (1995), 'Discourse analysis of the anti-female genital mutilation movement: Representation in western mainstream media.' *Commo/Oddities*: *A Journal of Communication and Culture,* July, Vol. 2 Pgs. 36-43

Hurst, Jane (1983), "The History of Abortion in the Catholic Church: The Untold Story", *Catholic for a Free Choice*, Washington, D.C.

Hussaina, A. (1995), 'Wifeism and Activism: The Nigerian Women's Movement.' *In The Challenges of Local Feminisms,* West View Press, Inc

Ilumoka, A. O. (1991), 'Policy and Law Relating to Abortion in Nigeria: The Quest for Balance' in Proceedings of seminar titled "Prevention of morbidity and mortality from induced and unsafe abortion in Nigeria" organized by the Department of Obstetric, Gynaecology and Perinatology; at Obafemi Awolowo University, Ile – Ife, Nigeria, Pgs. 113 - 124

Imam, A. (1994), "Politics, Islam and Women in Kano, Northern Nigeria." *Identifying Politics and Women*, Boulder: West-view Press.

Imam, Z. (1994), 'India bans female feticide', *British Medical Journal*, Vol. 309 (6952), Pg. 428

Imanyara, G. (ed.), 'Why Abortion is Reprehensible', *in The African Law Review*, Issue 72, Jun. 1998.

Inkeles, A. (1983), "Exploring Individual Modernity". New York: Columbia University Press.

International Conference of Human Rights; Tehran Proclamation, 1968.

International Family Planning Perspectives, 2001, Vol. 27(2), Pgs. 77-81

International Family Planning Perspectives, 2001, Vol. 27(3), Pgs. 144-147 & 151

International Planned Parenthood Federation, (1982), 'Adolescent Fertility and Family Planning: A Review of Selected Studies' London

Irvin, A. (2000), 'Taking Steps of Courage: Teaching About Sexuality and Gender in Nigeria and Cameroon.' *IWHC*

Irvine, J. M. (1990). 'Disorders of Desire: Sex and Gender in Modern American Sexology.' Philadelphia: Temple University Press.

Jacobson, J. L. (1990), ' The Global Politics of abortion' Washington, D.C. World Watch, Paper Number 97, July; Pg. 1-39

John, P. and Grisela, C. (1975), "Contraception and Family Design: A Study of Birth Planning in Contemporary Society." Edinburgh Press.

Johnson, D. (2000):'Abortion: The French Solution.' in *Post Express*, Feb. 24. Pg.12

Kakembo, Titus W. (1999), 'East Africa Tops Abortion Chart', in *The Monitor*, Feb. 3. Pg. 1

Kett, J. F. (1977), 'Rites of Passage: Adolescence in America, 1790 to the Present.' New York Book: Basic Books, in Craig et al. "Sociology", (1994).

Khan, S. et al. (1991), 'Effect on mortality of community based Maternity- Care program in Bangladesh.' *Lancet,* Vol. 338 (8776), Pgs. 1183-1186

Kisekka, M. et al. (1992), 'Determinants of Maternal Mortality in Zaria Area.' *In Women's Health Issues in Nigeria,* Jos: Tamaza Publishing Co., Pgs. 51 - 66.

----------, (1992), 'Women's Organized Health Struggles: The Challenge to Women's Organizations.' *Op. cit*, Pgs. 105 - 121

Kissling, F. (1999), 'Religion: Getting Involved' *in the Earth Times*, Hague, Feb. 6, Pgs. 2-6

Kluckhohn, C. (1960), 'The Concept of Culture.' *In Readings in Sociology*, ed. Schuler et al. Crowell Company New York.

Kosomo-Thomas, O. (1987) "The Circumcision of Women: A Strategy for Eradication." London: Dotesios Ltd.

Kamran, et al. (1979), "Controversies in Contraception." Wilkins Publishing.

Konje, J.C. et al. (1992), 'Health and economic consequences of septic induced abortion', *International Journal of Gynaecology and Obstetrics*, Vol. 37

Kramer, H. (1998), (ed) 'Changing Gender Culture: The U.S. Experience' by Sandra Lipsitz Bem, in Globalisation of Communication and Intercultural Experience, *Documentation of an International Conference* held on July 17-18, 1997 at the FU-Berlin, Pgs.107-121

Krieger, L.M. (1998), "RU 486 Abortion Pill Still not widely Available in the U.S." San Francisco Examiner, Jan. 27.

Ladipo, O.A. et al. (1986), 'Sexual behavior, contraceptive practice and reproductive health among Nigeria adolescents.' *Studies in Family Planning,* Vol. 17(2), Pgs. 100-106

Laurence, H.T. (1992), "Abortion: The Clash of the Absolutes", Norton W.W. & Company.

Lamnek, S. (1998), "Gruppendiskussion: Theorie und Praxis", Psychologie

Verlags Union, Weinheim.

Lightfoot-Klein, H. (1989), "Prisoners of Ritual: An Odyssey into Female Genital Circumcision in Africa." New York, Harrington Park Press

Lindsay, B. (1980), (ed.) "Comparative Perspectives of Third World Women: The Impact of Race, Sex and Class." Praeger Publishers, USA .

Linke, U. (1986), "AIDS in Africa." *Science* Vol. 231, Pg. 203

Lukumbo, L. (1998), 'Comments on Harmful Traditional Practices in Reproductive Health', *in Good Health Column, The Vanguard* Nov. 17, Pg.10

Lynn Thomas, (1998), "Imperial Concerns and 'Women's Affairs', State Efforts to Regulate Clitoridectomy and Eradicate Abortion in Meru, Kenya, 1910-1950," *Journal of African History,* Vol. 39(1), Pgs. 121-146

Madunagu, B. (1998), 'Adolescents: Taking Charge of their Sexuality.' MacArthur Foundation Newsletter, (2), Pgs. 10-11

Maendeleo Ya Wanawake Organization and the Program for Appropriate Technology in Health (1991), "Qualitative Research Report on Female Circumcision in Four Districts in Kenya." Nairobi: *Maendeleo Ya Wanawake Organization;* Pg. 18

Mandara, M. U. (1995), 'Procedure of female genital mutilation in Zaria: A critical Appraisal in Discussing Reproductive Rights in Nigeria', Rainbo.

Makinwa-Adebusoye, P. (1991), 'Contraception among urban Youth in Nigeria' Presented at the Demographic and Health surveys World Conference, Washington, D.C., Aug. 5 –7. Pg. 21

----------, (1992), 'Sexual Behaviour, Reproductive Knowledge and Contraceptive Use among Young urban Nigerians.' *International Family Planning Perspective,* Vol. 18(2), June, Pgs. 66 – 70

Malcolm, P & Wood, C. (1972), "New Concepts in Contraception" Oxford Med. & Technical Pub, Co. Pg. 231

Mannes, R. A. (1985), 'African practices may offer insights on AIDS.' *New York Times,* Nov. 22; and *in International Medicines,* Vol. 102, Pgs. 623-626

Maratmatsu, M. (1960), 'Effect of Induced Abortion on the Reduction of Birth in Japan' Milbank Memorial Fund Quarterly, 38, Pgs. 153-166

----------, (1977), 'Family Planning: History, Programmes and Practice' *In Population Problem Research Council, The Mainichi Newspaper, and the Japanese Organization for International Cooperation in Family Planning (JOICFP), eds. Fertility and Family Planning in Japan Tokyo, JOICFP,* Pgs, 21-51

Marx, P. (1998), "The Death Peddlers" Published by Human Life International (HLI), Australia Pgs. 1- 280

Marshall, G. (1998), "Oxford Dictionary of Sociology", Second Edition, Oxford University Press

Mba, M. (1982), "Nigerian Women Mobilized." Berkeley: International Studies, University of California

McCaffery, M. (1995), 'Management of female genital mutilation: The

Northwick Park Hospital experience.' *Journal of Obstetrics and Gynaecology,* Vol. 102, Pgs. 787-790

McCormick, E.P. (1975), "Attitudes towards abortion: Experience of Selected Black and White Women." Lexington Books.

McFarlane, D. R. (1993), "Induced Abortion: An Historical Overview", *American Journal of Gynaecologic Health,* Vol. VII, No. 3, May/June; Pgs. 77 82

McLean, S. (Ed.). (1980), "Female Circumcision, Excision and Infibulation: The Facts and Proposal for Change." London: Minority Rights Group.

Merton, R. K. (1960), 'Manifest and Latent Functions.' *In Readings in Sociology,* eds. Schuler et al. Crowell Company, New York.

----------, (1982), "The unintended consequences of purposive social action in Sociological Ambivalence." New York: Free Press

Michael, T. M. (1994), "Post Abortion Aftermath: A Comprehensive Consideration", Sheed & Ward

Ministry of Foreign Affairs - Danida. (1995), "Report from the Seminar on Female Genital Mutilation." Copenhagen: Axel Nielsen & Son.

Mohammad, R. (1999), 'Cultural and Social Dimension of FGM', "in Moving FORWARD", A report of the conference on female genital mutilation at the friends' house, London. Pgs. 2-5.

Mohamud, A.O. (1991), 'Female Circumcision and Child Mortality in urban Somalia' *Genus,* Vol. 47(3-4), Somalia, Pgs. 203-223

Mohr, J. (1978), "Abortion in America, New York". Oxford Univ. Press.

Mutenbei, I. B., and Mwesiga, M. K. (1998), 'The Impact of obsolete traditions on HIV/AIDS rapid transmission in Africa: The case of compulsory circumcision on young girls in Tanzania.' (Abstract. 23473), *International Conference on AIDS,* Vol.12, Pg. 436

Myers, R.A. et al. (1986), 'Circumcision: Its Nature and Practice Among Some Ethnic Groups in Southern States of Nigeria' *Social Sciences and Medicine,* Vol. 21(5), Pgs. 581-588

Nare, C. et al. (1997), 'Adolescents access to reproductive health and family planning services in Dakar (Senegal)' African Journal of Reproductive Health, Vol. 1(2), Pgs.15-24

Nasir, J. et al. (2000), 'Women Activist Criticize Constitution.' *The Guardian,* Jan 23.

National Population Commission, *Nigeria Demographic and Health Survey 1999.* Abuja, Nigeria: The Commission, 2000.

National Population Review, (1998), 'All Things Considered' *Transcript* H98052716: 212.

Neugarten, B. L., and Neugarten, D. A. (1987), 'The changing meanings of age.' *Psychology Today,* Vol. 21(5), Pgs.29-33

Nevadomsky, J. J. (1988), 'Ethics in Social Research', *Unpublished Monograph,* University of Benin, Nigeria Pgs.1-29

Nicholas, D. et al. (1986), 'Sexual Behaviour, Contraceptive Practice and Reproductive Health Among Nigerian Adolescents.' *Studies in Family Planning*, Vol. 18, No.3

Nigerian Tribune (1999), '1999 Constitution: Constitution of the Federal Republic of Nigeria.' Lagos. Pgs. 16-19

Nomboniso, Gasa-Suttner (1996), "The Empowerment of Women in South Africa" Pgs.18-20

Nunes, F.E. and Delph, (1997), 'Making Abortion Law Reform Work: Steps and Slips in Guyana' *Reproductive Health Matters*, No. 9 May. Pgs. 66-76

Obermeyer, Carla, Makhlouf (1994), "Religious Doctrine, State Ideology, and Reproductive options in Islam" *in Power and Decision: the Social Control of Reproduction,* Cambridge, M. A. Harvard School of Public Health, Pgs. 59-75

----------, (1994), 'Reproductive Choice in Islam: Gender and State in Iran and Tunisia' *Studies in Family Planning,* Vol. 25(1), Pgs. 41-51

Odoi-Agyarko, H. (1998), 'Harmful Traditional Practices in Reproductive Health: Packaging Population Advocacy and IEC by Journalists.' *In The Vanguard* (Good Health Column) Nov. 11, Pg. 10

Odujirin, O. (1991), 'Sexual Activity, Contraceptive Practice and Abortion among Adolescents in Lagos, Nigeria.' *International Journal of Gynaecology and Obstetrics,* Vol. 34(4), Pgs. 361-366

Ogedengbe, O.K. et al. (1992), 'Improving Abortion Care at the intermediated Level through Use of Manual Vacuum Aspiration: Results from Nigeria.' *Unpublished paper* presented at 32nd Annual Conference of the West African College of Surgeons, Banjul, Gambia, Feb. 2-9

Ogiamen, T. B.E. (1991), 'A legal framework to legalize abortion in Nigeria' *in Critical Issues in Reproductive Health,* Proceedings of seminar organized by the Department of Obstetrics and Gyneacology and Perinatology, O.A.U., Ile ife, Nigeria, December 4-6.

Ogunbunmi, K. (1999), 'Circumcision Helps Check HIV', *In The Guardian,* Dec. 26.

Ogwuda, A. (2000), 'Delta Moves Against Female Circumcision', *In The Vanguard,* Dec. 1.

Ojo, O.A. et al. (1994), 'An Evaluation of Provider Acceptability and Use of Manual Vacuum Aspiration (MVA) in Nigeria', *Unpublished Paper,* Pg. 15

Okagbue, I. (1990), 'Pregnancy Termination and the Law in Nigeria' *in Studies in Family Planning.* Vol. 21(4), July/Aug., Pgs. 196-209

Okojie, S. E. (1976), 'Induced Illegal Abortion in Benin City, Nigeria' *International Journal of Gynaecology and Obstetrics,* Vol. 14 (6), Pg. 517

Okonofua, F.E. et al. (1992), 'Illegal induced abortion: A study of 74 cases in Ile-Ife, Nigeria.' *Tropical Doctor,* Vol. 22, Pgs.75-78

Okonofua, F.E. (1999), 'HIV/AIDS Epidemic: call for a Pragmatic National Response', *Women's Health and Action Research Centre,* Vol. 4(2), Pg. 3

Okonofua, F.E. (1999), 'Infertility and reproductive health in Africa.' *African*

Journal of Reproductive Health, Vol. 3 (1), Pgs. 7 - 9

Okonofua, F.E. et al. (1999), 'Assessment of the health services for treatment of sexually transmitted infections among Nigerian adolescents', Sexually Transmitted Diseases, Vol. 26(3), Pgs. 184-190

Okumagba, M.P. (1982). "A Short History of the Urhobos." Kris and Pat, Nig. Ltd.

Oilkeh, A. (1981), "The place of sex education in secondary schools in Nigeria." *Nigerian School Health Journal,* Vol. 3(1), Pgs. 27-38

Oladipo, O. & Akintayo, T. (1991), 'Secondary school teacher's view point on sex education.', *Journal of the Royal Society of Health* Vol. 111, Pgs. 216-220

Olowu, F. (1998), 'Quality and cost of family planning as elicited by an adolescent mystery client trial in Nigeria' *African Journal of Reproductive health*, Vol. 12(1), pgs. 49-60

Olukoya, A.A. (1987), 'Pregnancy Termination: Results of a Community Based Study in Lagos, Nigeria', *International Journal of Gynaecology and Obstetrics*, Vol.25 (1), Pgs. 41- 46

Olukoya, P. (1996), "NGOs: Banding Together to Shape Policy in Nigeria." Mac Arthur Home Page, www.Mcarthur.com accessed on the 10/03/2002 at 4.00pm.

Olusanya, P. (1969), 'Nigeria: Cultural Barrier to Family Planning among the Yorubas.' *Studies in Family Planning*, Vol. 33, Pgs. 13-16

Omoigui, N. (2001), 'PROTEST AGAINST BILL H22 OUTLAWING FGM IN NIGERIA.' *Jenda: A Journal of Culture and African Women Studies*, Vol.1. Pg. 8.

Omorodion, F.I. (1998), 'Introduction to Social Research: The Nature of Surveys.' *Unpublished Monograph*, University of Benin Pgs. 12-17

Omorodion, F.I. and Myers, R.A. (1989), 'Reasons for female Circumcision Among some Ethnic Groups in Bendel State, Nigeria.' *African Study Monograph*, Vol. 9(4) Pgs.199-207

Omorodion, F.I. & Olusanya, O. (1998), 'The social context of reported rape City, Nigeria.' *The African Journal of Reproductive Health* Vol. 2(2), Pgs. 37-4

Omu, E. A. et al. (1981), 'Adolescent induced abortion in Benin City, *International Journal of Gynaecology and Obstetrics,* Vol. 19, Pgs. 495-499

Omu, S. (2000), 'Women in Power', Paper delivered at a confere "Parliamentarians for Global Action". Co-sponsored by, the Ford Founda United Nations Development Fund for Women (UNIFEM), UN, New York, U.! 9, Pg. 16

Onwuejeogwu, M.A. (2001), 'Women's reproductive health in traditional society: coping with human infertility and other maladies through the mecha marriage institutions among the Igbo of South – East Central Nigeria' Paper pre Seminar held at the Institut für Soziologie in the Freie Universität Berlir Germany, June 25 – July 2, 2001, Pgs. 3-53

Otite, & Ogionwon (1981), "An Introduction to Sociological Studies", Heinemann Educational Books (Nig.) Limited Pgs. 13-25

Otoide, V. (2000), 'Promoting Post - Abortion Care in Nigeria', *Women's Health and Action Research Centre,* Benin City, Nigeria, Vol. 5 (1), Pgs. 3-4

Otoide, V.O. et al. (2001), 'Why Nigerian adolescents seek Abortion rather than Contraception: Evidence From Focus Groups discussions.' *The International Family Planning Perspective* Vol. 27, Pgs. 77-81

Oyugi, C. (1998), 'Social Cultural Factors that Promote Female Circumcision and How this Predisposes Women to HIV Infection.' *International conference on AIDS,* Vol. (12) Pg. 1011-1012

Ozumba, B.C. (1992), 'Acquired gynetresia in Eastern Nigeria.' *International Journal of Gynaecology and Obstetrics,* Vol. 37, Pgs. 105-109

Palley, M.L. (1990), 'Women's Right as Human Rights: An International Perspectives', *Annals of American Academy of Political Science*, Vol. 515, Pgs, 163-178

Parsons, C. (1995), 'Guilt Over Abortion is Rare', The Globe and Mail, Sept. 14.

Passmore, S. L. (1981), "Against the Mutilation of Women: The Struggle to End Unnecessary Suffering." London: Ithaca.

Paul, B. (1993), 'Maternal mortality in Africa.' *Social Sciences Med.* Vol. 37, Pgs. 745-752.

Pcarce, T. (1993), 'The Country Strategy for the Population Program in Nigeria.' *Report Submitted,* to the MacArthur Foundation. Chicago.

----------, (1995), 'Health and Reproduction: Monitoring the Impact of Contraceptive Technology on Women in Nigeria' *Hay, T., and Stichter, S. (Eds.) African Women South of the Sahara*, Essex: Longman.

----------, (2001), 'Women, The State and Reproductive Health Issues in Nigeria.' *In Jenda*: ISSN 1530-5686

Pieters, G. (1972), 'Gynaecology au pays des femmes cousues' Acta Belgium, Vol. 71, Pgs. 173-193

Poley, M. (1983) "Contraception". London. Update Publication.

Population Action International (1994), "Financing the Future: Meeting the Demand for Family Planning; "A 1994 Report on Progress Towards World Population Stabilization"; Washington, D.C. ISSN: 0199-9761.

----------, (1997), "Contraceptive Choice: Worldwide Access to Family Planning; A 1997 Report on Progress Towards World Population Stabilization" Washington, D.C.

Population Council Report, (1991), "Prevention of Morbidity and Mortality for Unsafe Abortion, in Nigeria" NY: Population Council.

Population Crisis Committee (1991), "Access to Affordable Contraception:

1991 report on World Progress Towards Population Stabilization." Washington, D.C. ISSN: 0199-9761.
Population Reference Bureau (PRB) Inc 'The World's Youth 1996', *Health Issues* Washington, D. C. Pgs 1- 4
Prada, E. et al. (1989), 'Adolescents of Today, Parents of Tomorrow, Colombia' (SPA) *PROFAMILIA* Vol. 5(14), Pgs. 33-43
Probyn, E. (1992), 'Theorizing Through the Body.' In L. Rakow (Ed.), *"Women Making Meaning: New Feminist Directions in Communication"* New York: Routledge.
Qualls, Alyssa. (1990),"Women in Nigeria, Today." U.K.
Raspberry, W. (1993), 'Women and a Brutal Tradition.' *The Washington Post*, Nov. 8. Pg. A21
Rathmann, W.G. (1959), "Female Circumcision: indications and New Techniques" GP. Sept., Vol. XX (3), Pgs. 115-120
Rector, R. (1995) 'The Impact of New Jersey's Family Cap on Out – of Wedlock Births & Abortions.' *The Heritage Foundation,* FYI, No 59
Redfield, R. (1960), "A Critique of Cultural Relativism." *In Readings in Sociology,* eds. Schuler et al. Crowell Company, New York.
Reproductive Health Communication in Kenya (1994), 'The National Council for Population and Development and the John Hopkins University Population Communication Services (JHU/PCS) implemented the Kenya National Information, Education, and Communication Situation Survey (KNIECSS)' Chapters 8 and 9
Riley, M. W (1987), 'On the significance of age in sociology.' *American Sociological Review*, Feb. Vol. 52, Pgs. 1-14
Robert, Francoeus T. (1991), 'Biology, History, Politics of Abortion', Oklahoma, Dec. 28, Pgs. 1-3
Robinson, S. (2001), "The Last Rites." *In The Time Magazine,* Vol. 158 (23), Pgs.70-71
Rodney, W. (1974), "How Europe Underdeveloped Africa." Washington, D.C.: Howard University Press
Rosenthal, A. M. (1993c), 'Female Genital Torture.' *New York Times*, Dec. 29 Pg.A15
Rostow, W.W. (1960), "The Stages of Economic Growth, a non-communist manifesto." Cambridge University Press
Rothman, B. (1989), "Recreating Motherhood: Ideology and Technology in a Patriarchal Society." New York: Norton Publishing Company.
Rowe, P. J. (1985), 'Worldwide Patterns of infertility: Is Africa different?' *Lancet.* Vol. 2, Pgs. 596-598
Saltman, J. & Saltman, S. (1973), "Abortion Today." Zimmering Springfield.
Schaefer, R. T. (1997), "Social Policy and Gender Stratification: The Battle Over Abortion" McGraw-Hill
Schellenberg, J.A. (1996), "Conflict Resolution: Theory Research and

Practice", State University of New York Press

Seager, Joni et al, (1997), "State of Women in the World", 2nd edition, New York, Pengium Books

Shelton, J.D. (2001), 'The Provider Perspective: Human after all', *International Family Planning Perspectives*, Vol. 27(3), Pgs. 152-153

Schuler, H. et al. (1960), "Readings in Sociology." Second edition Thomas Y. Crowell Company. U.S.A.

Shlomo, A. (1968), "The Social and Political Thought of Karl Marx", Cambridge University Press

Shyma, T. and Saraswati, M.P. (2001), 'Induced abortion in urban Nepal', *International Family Planning Perspectives*, Vol. 27(3), Pgs. 144-147

SIECUS International Program, (1995) 'Training for Sexuality Education' *in AHI's GROWING UP*, Dec., Vol. 3(4)

----------, (1996), 'A Call for Action' *in AHI's GROWING UP*. Vol. 4(2.)

----------, (1996), "Preventing HIV/AIDS: Teens Learn Risk Reduction Skills", *Action Health Incorporated*, Sept. Vol. 4(3.)

----------, (1997), 'SIECUS report: Abstinence-only education, SIECUS, April/May, Vol. 25(4), Pg. 16

Steady, F. C. (1990), 'Women: The Gender Factor in the African Social Situation.' ACARTSOD. London.

Stockdale, J. (1996), 'The Threat of HIV: Coping with Condoms', Economic and Political Sciences. *LSE magazine.*

Swindler, A. (1986), 'Culture in action: Symbols and strategies' *In American Sociological Review* Vol. 51, Pgs. 273-286

Tietze, C. and Lewit, S. (1972), 'Joint Programme for the study of Abortion (JPSA): Early medical complications of Legal abortion', *Studies in Family Planning,* 3(6), Pgs. 97-119

The Awake Magazine (1993),'The Abortion Dilemma: Are 60 million killings the Solution.' May 22, Pgs. 3 - 9.

----------, (1992), 'How Bad AIDS is in Africa', Aug. 8, Pgs. 3-11

----------, (1994), 'Helping Those With AIDS', Mar. 22, Pgs. 12- 15

----------, (1996), 'More Abortions in Canada', Feb. 22. Pgs 28

The International Development Magazine, (1999), 'Developments: Let's Talk About Sex', Issue 6, Second Quarter, Pgs. 26-27

The Nigerian Demographic and Health Survey, 1990. Pgs. 1-25

The Society of Gynaecology and Obstetrics of Nigeria (SOGON) memorandum to the Federal Government of Nigeria (1974)

Thevoz, M. (1984), "The Painted Body" New York: Rizzoli International Publishing Incorporated.

Todaro, M.P. (1982), "Economics For A Developing World." Second Edition, Long-man Group Ltd. U.K.

Toubia, N. (1993), "Female Genital Mutilation: A Call for Global Action." New York: Women, Ink.

----------, (1994), 'Female circumcision as a public health measure.' *International English Journal of Medicine,* Vol. 331, Pgs. 712-716

----------, **(1994),** 'FGM and Responsibility of Reproductive Health Professionals.' *International Journal Gynaecology & Obstetrics*, Vol. 46, Pgs, 127-135

Toubia, N. and Bulut, A. (1994), 'Efficiency and Effectiveness of Public Sector Abortion Services in Istanbul and their Suitability to Women's Needs.' Istanbul and New York, University of Istanbul and Population Council, Pg. 21

Tumachine, D. (1978), "Unwanted Pregnancy- accident or illness?" Oxford University, Press

United Nations (1989), 'Adolescent Reproductive Behaviour - Evidence from Developing Countries' Vol. II. New York.

----------, (1991), 'United Nations Proposes Action to Prohibit Violence Against Women', *UN Chronicle* 28, Pgs. 68-69

----------, (1994), 'Population and Development: Programme of Action Adopted at the International Conference on Population and Development', Cairo, Sept. 5-13, Vol. 1, New York: United Nations Department for Economic and Social Information and Policy Analysis

----------, (1995), 'Report of the Fourth World Conference on Women', Beijing Sept. 4-15. New York: United Nations.

UNAIDS (1998), 'The Public Health Approach to STD Control.' Technical Update, Pgs. 3-7

----------, (1999), ' HIV/AIDS: Emerging Issues and Challenges for Women, Young People and Infants.' Second Edition, Pgs. 11-16

----------, (1999), 'World AIDS Campaign: Facts and Figures', Joint United Nations Programme on HIV/AIDS (UNAIDS), Geneva Pgs. 5-8

UNDP/UNFPA/WHO/World Bank Special Program of Research, Development and Research Training in Human Reproduction: *Biennal Report* 1994-1995.

United Nations Children's Fund (1994), *Gender Equality and Women's Empowerment: A UNICEF Training* Package; New York: UNICEF

----------, (1994), 'Guideline for UNICEF action on eliminating female genital mutilation (Memorandum from James P. Grant, Executive Director.) *Unpublished document,* Oct. 31, Pg. 10

United Nations Development Program, (UNDP) report of baseline "Survey of Positive and Harmful Traditional Practices Affecting Women and Girls in Nigeria" (1997), Pg. 7

United Nations General Assembly (UNGA.) Universal Declaration of Human Rights, G.A. 217A (III), Dec.10, 1948; Human Rights: A Compilation of International Instruments. New York and Geneva: United Nations, 1994. Articles 1, 3, 19, 25 (1) and (2), 27

----------, Convention on the Elimination of All Forms of Discrimination Against Women, G.A. Res. 34/180, Dec. 18, 1979 (entered into force September 3, 1981.) Human Rights: A Compilation of International

Instruments; New York and Geneva:
United Nations 1994. Articles 10(h), 11(f), 12(1) and (2)
----------, Programme of Action of the international Conference on Population and Development. Doc. A/171/13, New York, October 18, 1994
----------, (1995), Beijing Declaration and Platform for Action: Fourth world Conference on Women, Doc A/Conf. 177/20, New York, Oct. 17
United Nations Population Information Network (UNPOPIN), UN Population Division, Department of Economic and Social Affairs, With Support from the UN Population Fund (UNFPA), "Reproductive Health and Family Planning, Technical Report 31", UNFPA, New York, Dec. 1994. Pgs. 8-9
Unuigbe, J. A. et al. (1988), 'Abortion - related morbidity and mortality in Benin City, Nigeria: 1973-1985.' *International Journal, of Gynaecology and Obstetrics,* Vol. 26(3), Pgs. 435-439
U.S. Agency for International Development Office of Women in Development (1996), USAID Gender Plan of Action: Bringing Beijing home. *Gender Action, Vol. 1(1),* Pg. 3
Verzim, J. A. (1975), ,Sequelae of female circumcision' Trep. Doct. Vol. 5, Pgs. 163-169
Victoria, I. (1999), 'Abortion: Report lists measures against scourge', *Daily Champion* Publication. Pg. 14
Waris, D. & Miller, C. (1998), "Desert Flower: The Extraordinary Journey of a Desert Normad." William Morrow.
Watters, Wendells W. (1976), "Compulsory Parenthood: The Truth about Abortion" McClelland and Stewart, Toronto.
Wernet, A. (2000), "Einführung in die Interpretationstechnik der Objektiven Hermeneutik", Leske + Budrich; Opladen.
Wolf-Dieter, J. (1982), 'The World as a Trading Place - On Cultural Proposition and Effect of the Lome Convention' *in IFDA,* Dossier 28, March – April. Pgs. 59
Women's Health Forum, (1997), 'Need to Address Adolescent Reproductive Health in Nigeria.' *Women's Health and Action Research Centre, Nigeria,* Vol, 2(2), ISSN 118-185XI, Pgs. 1-14
World Health Organization (1975), 'Pregnancy and abortion in adolescence: Report of WHO meeting.' Geneva. *WHO Technical report series* Nr. 583 Pg. 27
----------, (1979), 'Induced abortion guidelines for the provision of care and services.' Geneva, Pg. 69
World Health Organization, (1982), 'Oral Contraception; Technical and Safety Aspects.' Geneva, Pg. 45
----------, (1994), 'Contraceptives Method Mix: Guidelines for Policy and Service Delivery.' Geneva.
----------, (1993), 'Prevention and Management of Unsafe Abortion: Report of a Technical Working Group.' Geneva

----------, (1995), 'Female genital mutilation: Report of WHO Technical Working Group' Geneva: World health Organization, Pg. 9

WHON. (1996), 'Gender Based Violence - A violation of Human Rights, and an Affront to Women's Health.' Vol. 3(2), Pgs. 1-7

Yomere, G. & Agbonifoh, B. (1999), "Research Methodology in Social Sciences and Education", University of Benin, Press.

Zitner, A. (1997) 'The RU- 486 Saga', The Boston Globe. Nov.23.

NEWS ON-LINE:

www.Aghadiuno.com: accessed on the 22/03/2001 at 2.30 GMT

www.deltastate.org: accessed on the 30/05/2001 at 3.45 GMT

www.digitalrag.com/ai/womensrights/africa3.html: (Amnesty International), accessed on the 15/02/2002 at 1.21 GMT

www.bbc.co.uk: (News on Africa) accessed on the, 12/04/1998, 29/11/1999, and 5/04/2000 at 15.22, 18.00 and 9.41 GMT respectively

www.ngrguardiannews.com: accessed on the, 19/09/1999, 30/01/2000 29/02/2000, 10/06/2000, 1/07/2001 and 9/03/2001 at 15.00, 18.00, 1.30, 4.20, 7.15, and 18.45 GMT respectively

www.vanguardngr.com: accessed on the, 27/01/2000, 26/06/2000 and 9/03/2001 at 10.00, 3.32 and 12.45 GMT respectively

Casimir Chinedu O. Nzeh

From Clash to Dialogue of Religions

A Socio-Ethical Analysis of the Christian-Islamic Tension in a Pluralistic Nigeria

Frankfurt/M., Berlin, Bern, Bruxelles, New York, Oxford, Wien, 2002.
423 pp., num. fig. and tab.
European University Studies: Series 23, Theology. Vol. 745
ISBN 3-631-39350-4 · pb. € 60.30* / US $ 53.95 / £ 37.–
US-ISBN 0-8204-5969-0

September 11, 2001 is now etched into the collective world consciousness as a water-shed in the modern history of relationship between the world civilizations. These civilizations are essentially rooted in religious faiths that are largely ignorant of each other and consequently mutually hostile. Hopefully, not too late, the world has woken up to this awesome reality. This work started by the author some years ago before September 11, 2001 is appearing at a most auspicious time, when Nigeria indeed, is like the world-stage in microcosm where the contradictions between faith and praxis in the relationship between these world religions are played out. Using Nigeria as a case-study the author painstakingly analyses the commonly shared areas of faith between Islam and the Christian Faith and carefully too scrutinizes the background, motives and characteristics of the friction points between the two religions. The result of his research challenges both religions by exposing how much they have in common to co-exist peacefully and assure humanity that peace is inexorably bound up with religion. It also underscores the Catholic Social Teaching with its principles, values and norms for the foundation of a sound social Order and structure of social life.

Frankfurt/M · Berlin · Bern · Bruxelles · New York · Oxford · Wien
Distribution: Verlag Peter Lang AG
Moosstr. 1, CH-2542 Pieterlen
Telefax 00 41 (0) 32 / 376 17 27

*The €-price includes German tax rate
Prices are subject to change without notice
Homepage http://www.peterlang.de